Differential Diagnosis
in Pediatric Dermatology

Ernesto Bonifazi

Differential Diagnosis in Pediatric Dermatology

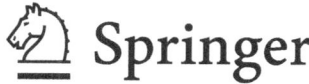 Springer

Ernesto Bonifazi
Dermatologist
Bari, Italy

This volume is based on the Italian edition released in 2012, with the author's and the publisher's authorization.

ISBN 978-88-470-3934-6
DOI 10.1007/978-88-470-2859-3

ISBN 978-88-470-2859-3 (eBook)

Springer Milan Heidelberg New York Dordrecht London

Cover design: Ikona S.r.l., Milano

Typesetting: Ikona S.r.l., Milano

Springer-Verlag Italia S.r.l. – Via Decembrio 28 – I-20137 Milan
Springer is a part of Springer Science+Business Media (www.springer.com)

To Carlo Meneghini,
unforgettable teacher

Foreword

Pediatric dermatology is the branch of dermatology that has acquired its own autonomous standing within the field of dermatology for many reasons. First, it is because of specific childhood diseases, such as neonatal dermatoses and Gianotti–Crosti and staphylococcal scalded skin syndrome. Then, there are those diseases that are typical, if not exclusive, of this age (atopic dermatitis, impetigo), those diseases that manifest themselves with different characteristics in the adult and child (dermatomyositis, psoriasis), and finally, those diseases that start in childhood but continue into adulthood (genodermatoses). Therefore, the approach to this fascinating but difficult discipline requires sound dermatological knowledge combined with pediatric sensitivity. For all these reasons, and for the frequency with which physicians encounter skin disorders in their daily clinical practice, more and more pediatricians are turning to it. This book is meant for them and for many dermatologists for whom pediatric dermatology has not been the main interest. The author is well known: Ernesto Bonifazi has long been a leading light and teacher of pediatric dermatology both in Italy and internationally. Readers of the *European Journal of Pediatric Dermatology*, the official journal of the European Society for Pediatric Dermatology, of which Ernesto was the second President, already know and value his column on differential diagnosis published in the journal. Such work reveals two main talents: his passion for teaching, which he has long exercised as Professor at the University of Bari and which manifests itself as a natural, clear, and concise exposition, and his experience, which is the result of many years of penetrating and precise clinical observations. The differential diagnoses are presented in pairs, concisely, and are accompanied by illustrative and coherent images. The book is an essential tool, a true distillation of practical dermatological knowledge. Consider this book as a good but discreet friend, though as valuable as only true friends can be.

Mauro Paradisi
Past President of the Italian Society
of Pediatric Dermatology

Preface

An original column dedicated to the differential diagnosis of skin diseases in children was consistently included in the Italian journal devoted to Pediatric Dermatology (*Pediatric Dermatology News*), which was founded in 1982 simultaneously with the American (*Pediatric Dermatology*) and Japanese (*Journal of Pediatric Dermatology*) journals, and changed its name in *European Journal of Pediatric Dermatology* in 1991.

The book you hold in your hand is a collection of all published differential diagnoses, plus others, revisited in the light of current clinical experience and accompanied by new images. Each chapter, which consists of two pages, refers to the differential diagnosis between two dermatological conditions (in exceptional cases, three or four), and contains 2–6 images and a very short text that emphasize the clinical differences between the two diseases. At the end of each chapter, a summary highlights one or two diagnostic characteristics essential for the differential diagnosis. The book should be of help to the growing number of physicians—pediatricians, dermatologists, general practitioners—interested in pediatric dermatology.

Ernesto Bonifazi

Acknowledgements

I would like to thank the following people: Mariella, who was responsible for the graphic design of the Italian edition of the book; Lucretia, who in the 35 years that we have worked together suggested, not infrequently, the themes for the chapters of the differential diagnoses; Vittorio, whose pertinent and penetrating questions got me to come back with answers that were often not that easy to find; Dino, who was always available and helped me deal with all the issues related to the publication of the book and was involved in proofreading it; Ilaria, for helping out with the photocomposition of the Italian edition; Antonella, who was always ready to provide a helping hand, and especially for the enthusiasm she put into contacting the children and their parents; and Paul, who helped photograph each child, a skill that is more difficult than you might imagine.

Moreover, my thanks go to Mario Cutrone, who provided the photos of streptococcal scarlet fever, and Tani Scanni for the photos of keratin hair casts and pubic lice.

Finally, I would like to thank all my friends, who like me dedicated their life to pediatric dermatology, particularly Iria who suggested the differential diagnosis between Spitz nevus and juvenile xanthogranuloma.

Contents

Inherited Skin Disorders

E. Bonifazi, *Differential Diagnosis in Pediatric Dermatology,*
DOI: 10.1007/978-88-470-2859-3_1 © Springer-Verlag Italia 2013

1. Neurofibromatosis
2. Macular Mastocytosis

Café au lait spots can be the only clinical sign of neurofibromatosis in babies. Macular mastocytosis can be characterized by brownish maculae simulating peripheral neurofibromatosis.

	1. Neurofibromatosis	2. Macular Mastocytosis
Definition	Autosomal dominant inherited disease, initially characterized by café au lait spots.	Benign proliferation of dermal mastocytes clinically characterized by brownish maculae.
Family history	Present in 30% of cases [1].	Present in 3% of cases [2].
Time of onset	Often present at birth or in the first months.	Mastocytosis is sometimes present at birth. It becomes evident in the first months of life.
Sites involved	Anywhere on the skin.	Mainly on the chest.
Darier sign	Absent.	Present, although barely evident due to the paucity of mastocytes.
Involvement of the groin region and axillary folds	Frequent.	Rare.
Lesion size	Highly variable, even within the same subject; larger lesions can exceed 5 cm; the smallest may measure less than 5 mm.	Rather uniform, usually 1–2 cm in diameter.
Lesion outline	Clearly defined.	Blurred.
Development	New lesions, usually smaller, appear with age. Pre-existing lesions usually persist unchanged.	No new lesions appear after the first year. Pre-existing lesions disappear in several years.

Diagnostic Summary

Neurofibromatosis: maculae of variable size with well-defined borders throughout the skin.

Macular mastocytosis: maculae with blurred borders mainly on the chest, which undergo slight urtication when rubbed.

1. Neurofibromatosis

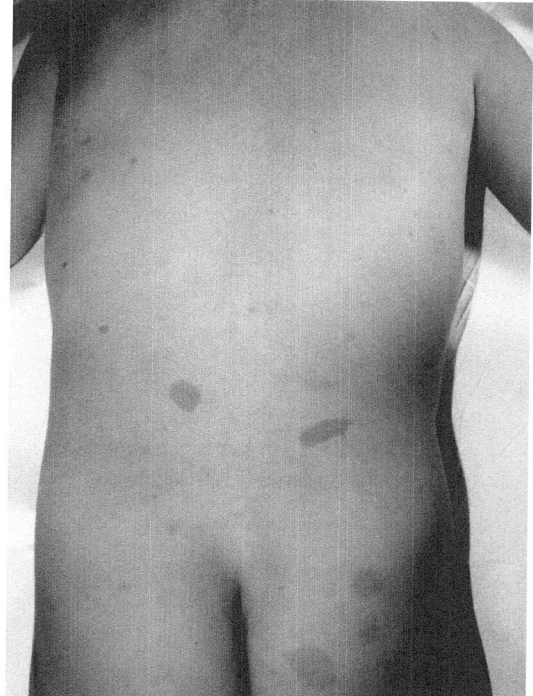

Fig. 1

2. Macular Mastocytosis

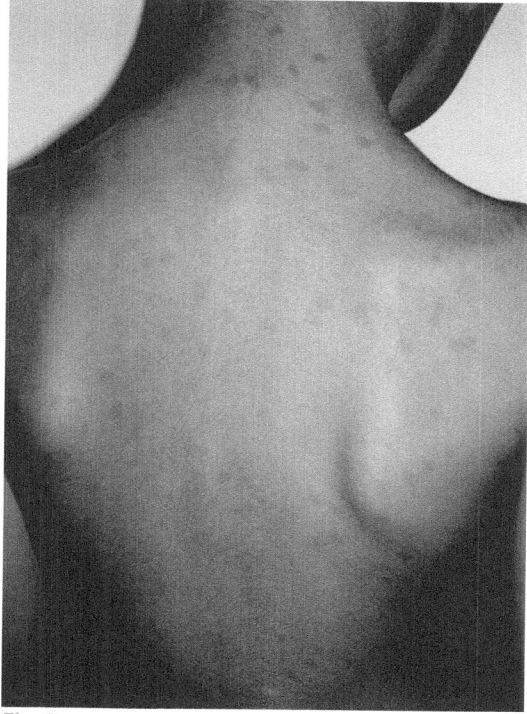

Fig. 2

1. Recessive Dystrophic Epidermolysis Bullosa
2. Bullous Congenital Ichthyosiform Erythroderma
   (Epidermolytic Hyperkeratosis)

Recessive dystrophic epidermolysis bullosa and bullous congenital ichthyosiform erythroderma can be present at birth with bullous lesions, particularly at sites of trauma, and thus require a differential diagnosis.

	1. Recessive Dystrophic Epidermolysis Bullosa	2. Bullous Congenital Ichthyosiform Erythroderma
Definition	Inherited disease due to a collagen defect, with consequent post-traumatic blisters and dystrophic scars.	Inherited disease due to a keratin defect, with consequent blisters and scaling erythroderma.
Heredity	Autosomal recessive.	Autosomal dominant.
Blood blisters	Often present.	Lacking.
Blister distribution	Hands, feet, elbows, knees.	Trunk, limbs.
Mouth blisters	Often present.	Lacking.
Generalized erythema	Lacking.	Present.
Healing of blisters	Slow, with milia and scarring.	Rapid, without scarring.

Diagnostic Summary

Recessive dystrophic epidermolysis bullosa: blisters at sites of trauma, also in the oral mucosa, sometimes hematic, arising on skin initially nonerythematous.

Bullous congenital ichthyosiform erythroderma: superficial blisters on erythematous and scaling skin, sparing the mucosae.

1. Recessive Dystrophic Epidermolysis Bullosa

2. Bullous Congenital Ichthyosiform Erythroderma

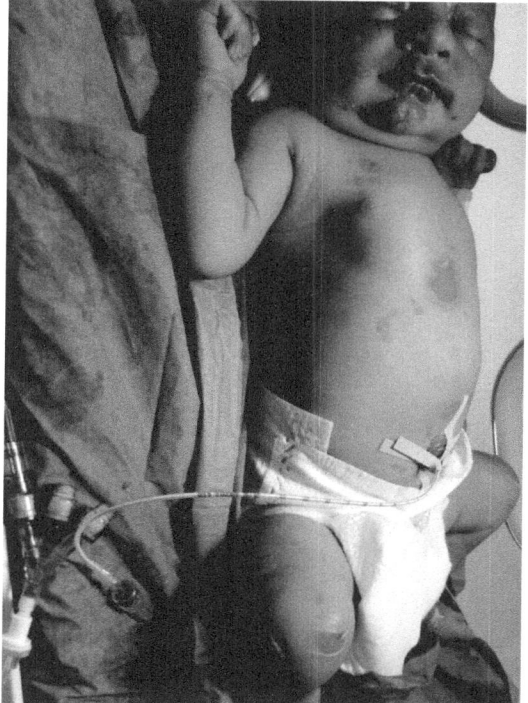

Fig. 1a

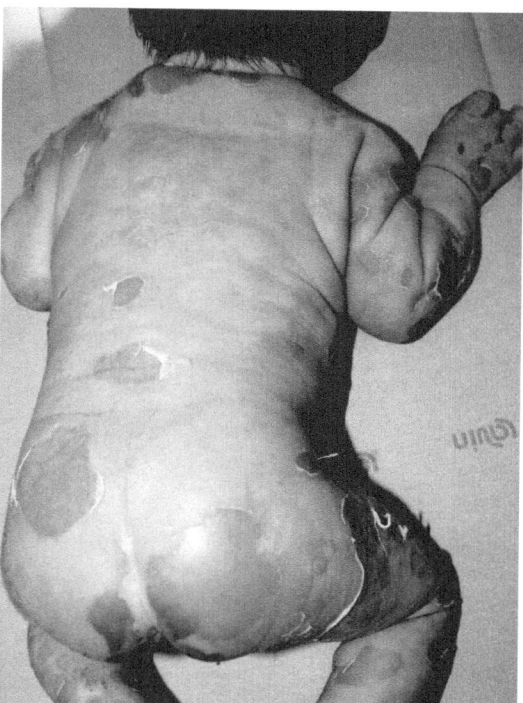

Fig. 2a

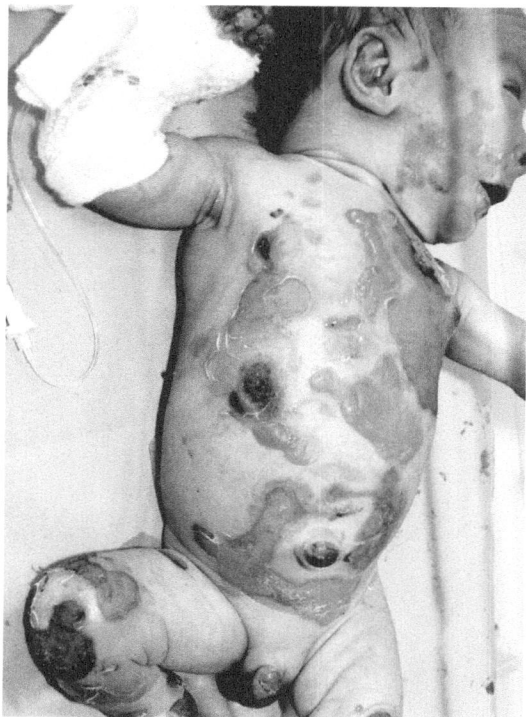

Fig. 1b Same newborn as in Fig. 1a, 10 days later

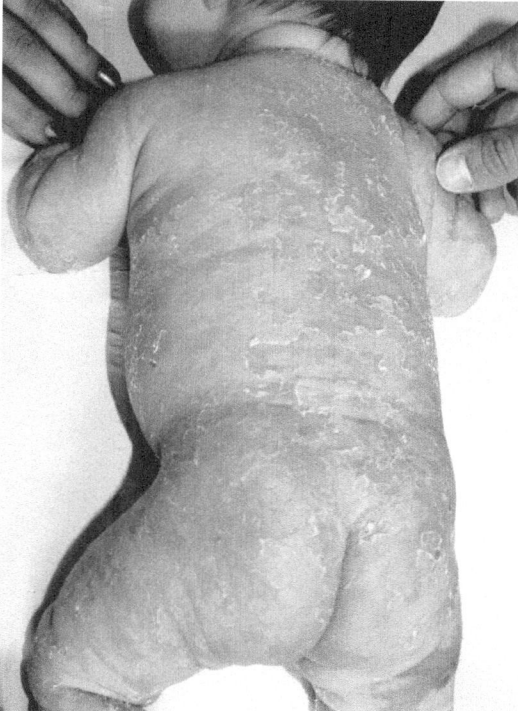

Fig. 2b Same newborn as in Fig. 2a, taken 10 days later

E. Bonifazi, *Differential Diagnosis in Pediatric Dermatology,*
DOI: 10.1007/978-88-470-2859-3_2 © Springer-Verlag Italia 2013

1. Aplasia Cutis Congenita
2. Sebaceous Nevus in the Newborn

The two most frequent causes of localized alopecia in the newborn are aplasia cutis and a sebaceous nevus. In the former, the lack of hair is due to the scarring of the healing process, whereas in the latter, it is due to hypertrophy of the sebaceous glands, which compress the hair, making it thinner.

	1. Aplasia Cutis Congenita	2. Sebaceous Nevus in the Newborn
Definition	Congenital, localized absence of epidermis, dermis and sometimes subcutaneous tissue, which heals with scarring.	Nevus with prominent involvement of the sebaceous glands.
Number of lesions	Usually single, sometimes multiple.	Usually only one.
Lesion morphology	Eroded or already scarred at birth. In the latter, the surface is smooth.	Granular.
Clinical course	At birth it presents already with a scarred appearance or as an erosion, sometimes crusted, that heals in a few days with residual scar or more rarely as a blister. The scar remains unchanged over time.	Usually present at birth, a sebaceous nevus does not change significantly until puberty. At this age, it often thickens due to hyperplasia of the sebaceous glands. Almost always benign tumors of adnexal origin may develop from the second decade [3].

Diagnostic Summary

Aplasia cutis congenita: smooth surface.

Sebaceous nevus in the newborn: granular surface.

1. Aplasia Cutis Congenita

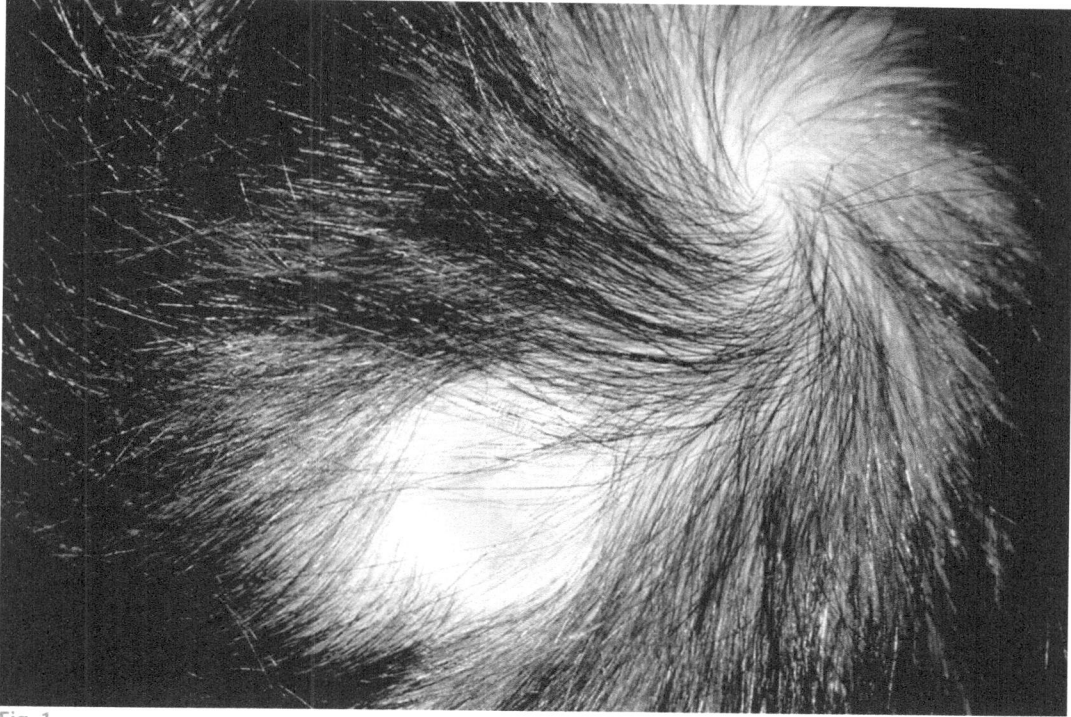

Fig. 1

2. Sebaceous Nevus in the Newborn

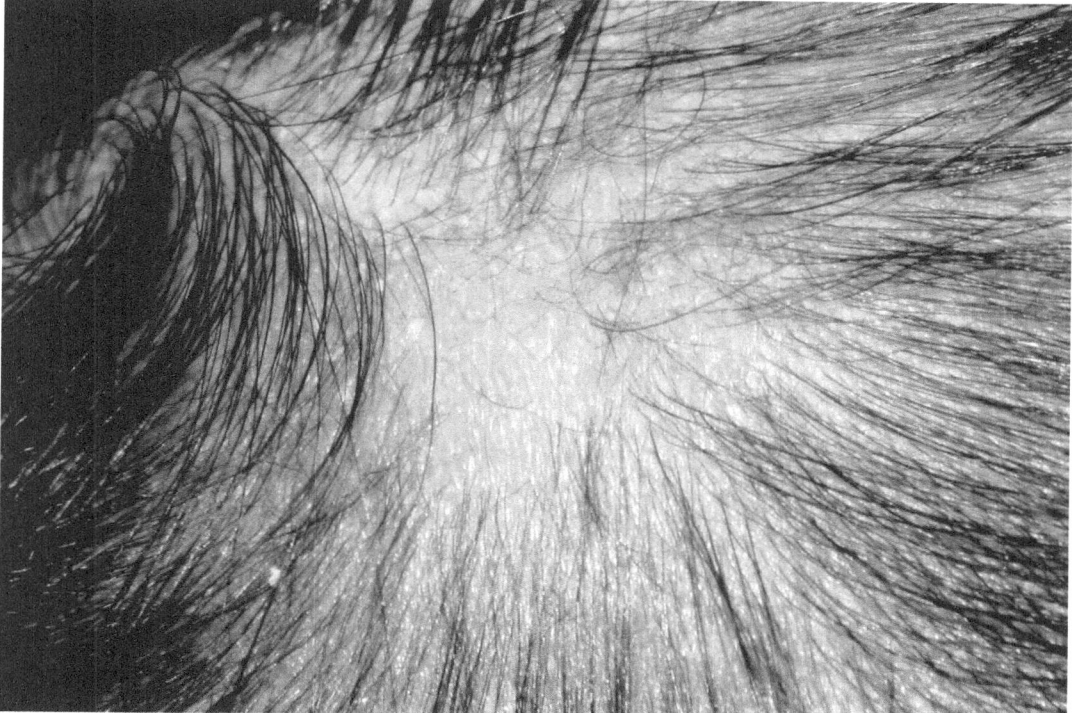

Fig. 2

1. Port-Wine Stain
2. Segmental Hemangioma

When present at birth, a hemangioma is flat; when extensive, it is often characterized by a segmental distribution, making it difficult to provide a differential diagnosis between port-wine stain and segmental hemangioma.

	1. Port-Wine Stain	2. Segmental Hemangioma
Presence at birth	As a rule.	In 50% of cases.
Small bulges	Absent.	Frequent after the first weeks.
Capillaroscopy	Dilated papillary and subpapillary plexus [4].	Desert papillary plexus, irregularly dilated subpapillary plexus.
Uniformity of color	Yes.	No.

Diagnostic Summary

Port-wine stain: uniform color, thin telangiectases and small bulges absent.

Segmental hemangioma: non-uniform color, often thin telangiectasias and, after a few weeks, small bulges.

1. Port-Wine Stain

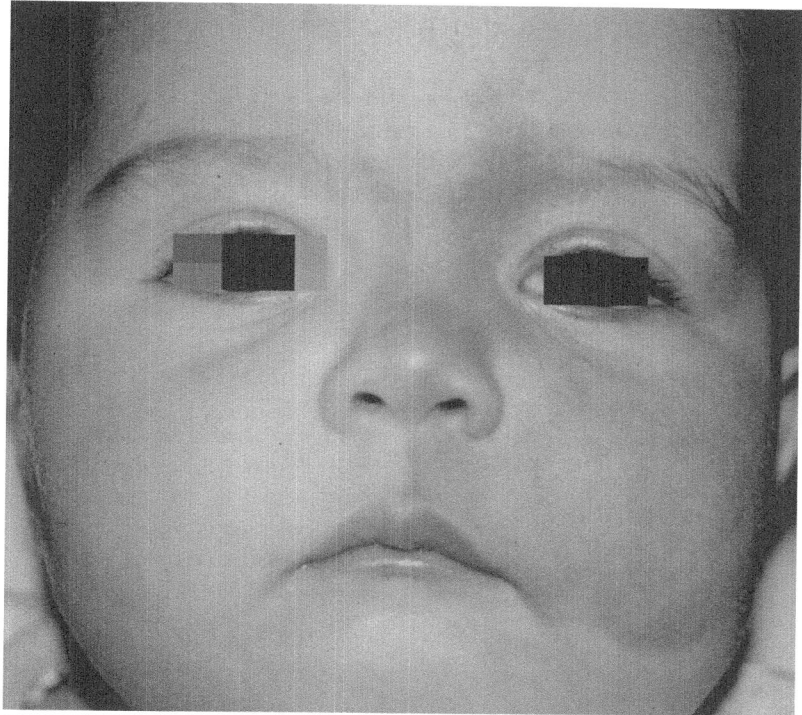

Fig. 1

2. Segmental Hemangioma

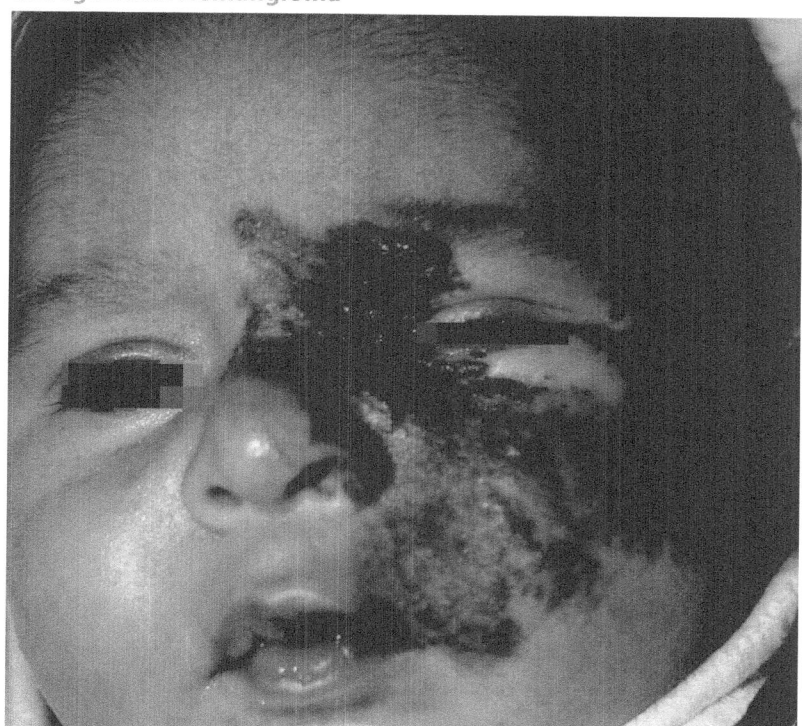

Fig. 2

1. Port-Wine Stain
2. Cutis Marmorata Telangiectatica Congenita

In the first days of life, making a differential diagnosis between port-wine stain (PWS) and cutis marmorata telangiectatica congenita (CMTC) can be difficult. Making a differential diagnosis between the two disorders is important, because the prognosis of PWS is more severe due to the higher frequency of associated malformations and the possible progressive deterioration, unlike CMTC which tends to improve with time.

	1. Port-Wine Stain	2. Cutis Marmorata Telangiectatica Congenita
Definition	Capillary malformation.	Complex vascular anomaly clinically characterized by an erythematous and cyanotic cutaneous reticulum, telangiectasias, phlebectasias, and ulceration in severe cases.
Frequency	About 1:500 newborns [5].	About 1:2,650 newborns [5].
Associated malformations	Possible and involving the central nervous system, eye, and the deep tissues of a limb.	Rare.
Facial involvement	Frequent in both segmental and generalized form.	Exceptional.
Lesion morphology	Erythematous-vinous, homogeneous, sometimes reticular appearance with thin mesh; never necrosis or ulceration.	Reticulum with large, erythematous, and cyanotic meshes, sometimes necrosis and ulceration, mainly at the level of the knee.
Clinical course	PWS remains unchanged over time, sometimes thickens on the face causing dental and gum alterations; possible appearance of eruptive angiomas.	CMTC never worsens with time, rather, it shows progressive improvement.

Diagnostic Summary

Port-wine stain: it often affects the face, is characterized by homogeneous erythematous-vinous patches and does not improve with time.

Cutis marmorata telangiectatica congenita: it does not affect the face, is characterized by a cyanotic reticulum with large meshes, and tends to improve with time.

1. Port-Wine stain

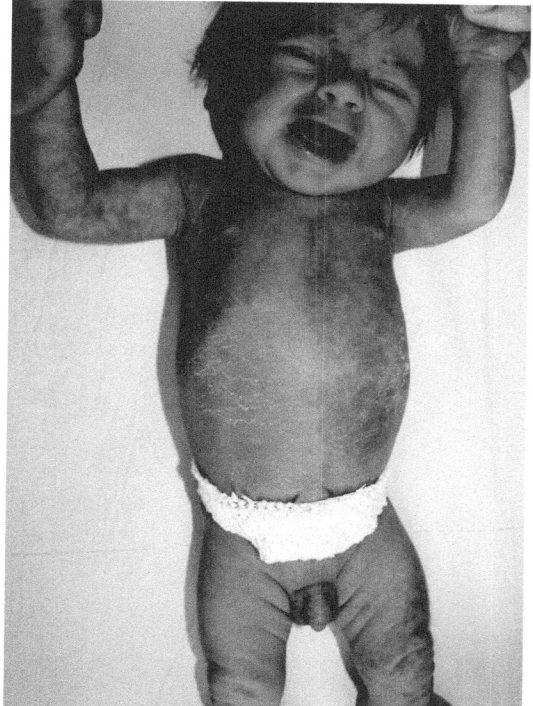

Fig. 1a

2. Cutis Marmorata Telangiectatica Congenita

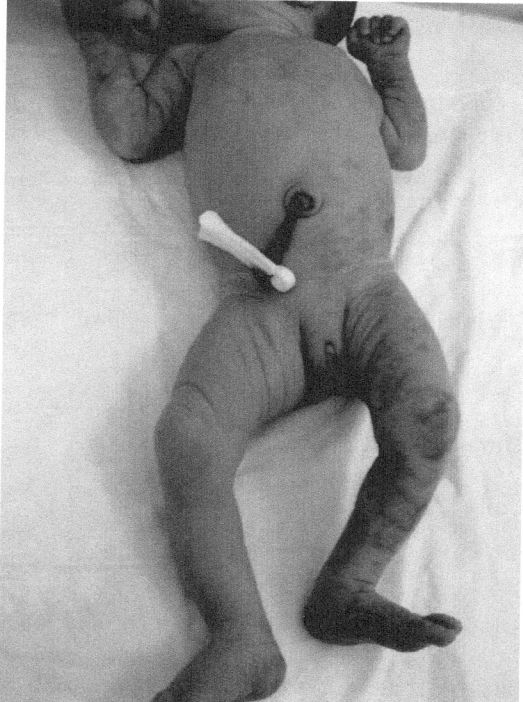

Fig. 2a

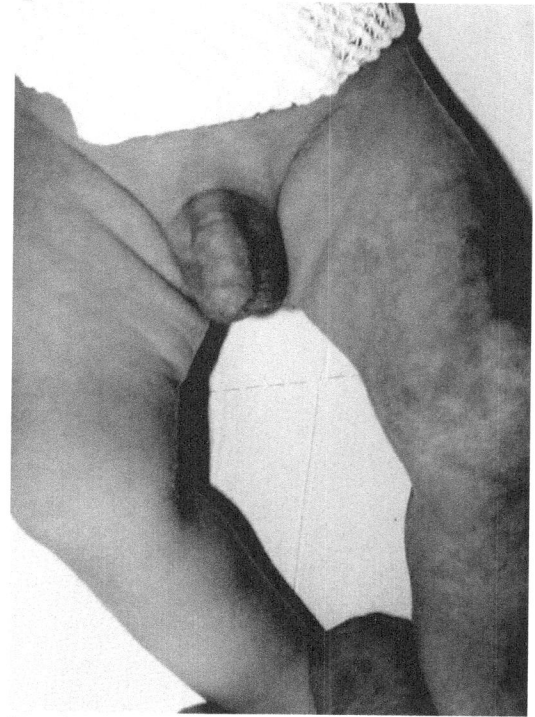

Fig. 1b

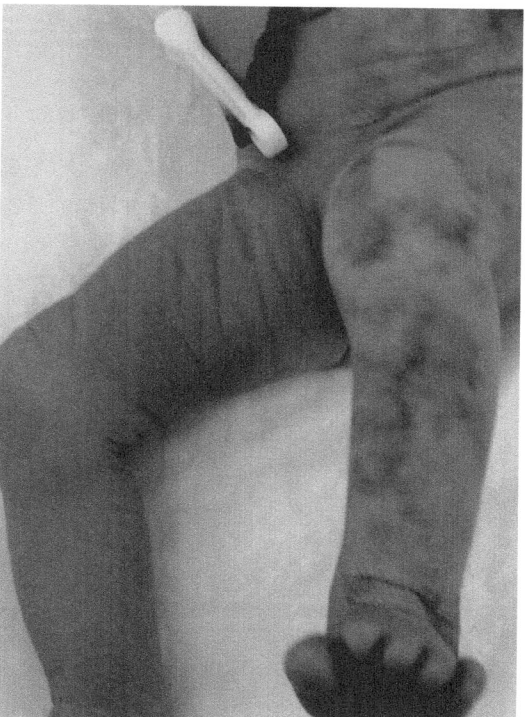

Fig. 2b

1. Pyogenic Granuloma
2. Hypopigmented Spitz Nevus

In children, a Spitz nevus is barely pigmented or unpigmented and looks like an angioma. This is why it is confused with and should be differentiated from pyogenic granuloma.

	1. Pyogenic Granuloma	2. Hypopigmented Spitz Nevus
Definition	Benign neoplasia of angiopoietic cells.	Benign neoplasia of spindle or epithelioid melanocytes with little pigmentation.
Time of onset	At any age.	Usually in the first decade of life.
Color	Usually red.	Red or red-brown. Under finger pressure, the brown pigmentation becomes more evident.
Shape	Hemispherical or lobular.	Hemispherical.
Base	Often pedunculated.	Sessile.
Epidermis	Initially intact, it erodes after a few weeks.	Usually intact.
Clinical course	It grows very rapidly (in a matter of weeks).	It grows rapidly (in a matter of months).
Bleeding	Yes, 3–4 weeks after its first appearance.	No [6].
Dermoscopy	Large vasal lacunae, with lobular appearance.	Dot-like vessels, regularly distributed in the center of whitish polygonal areas.

Diagnostic Summary

Pyogenic granuloma: it reaches its maximum size within 1 month and then bleeds.

Hypopigmented Spitz nevus: it reaches its maximum size within 6 months and does not bleed.

1. Pyogenic Granuloma

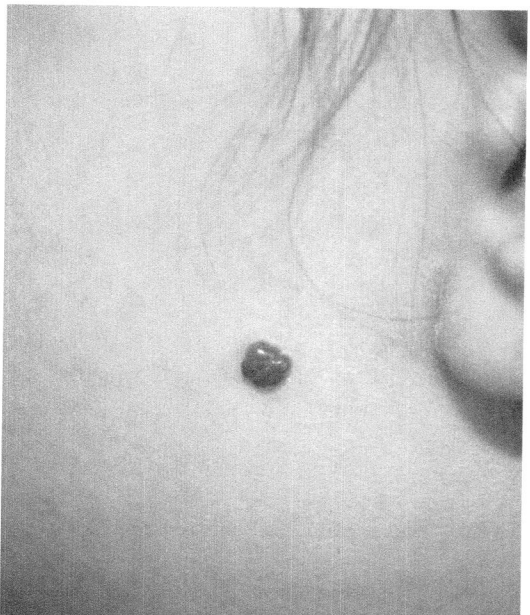

Fig. 1a

2. Hypopigmented Spitz Nevus

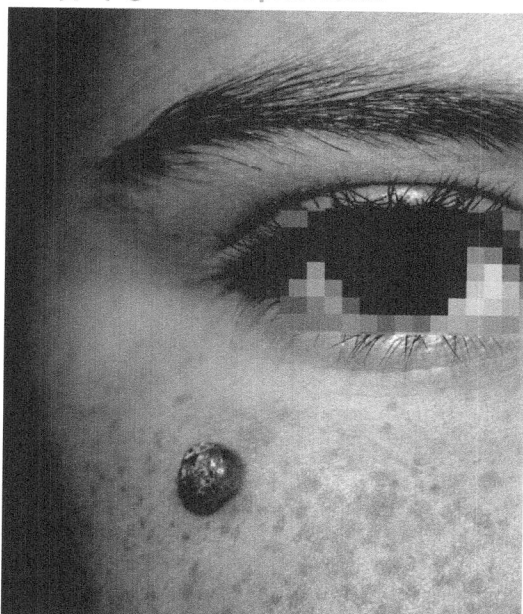

Fig. 2a

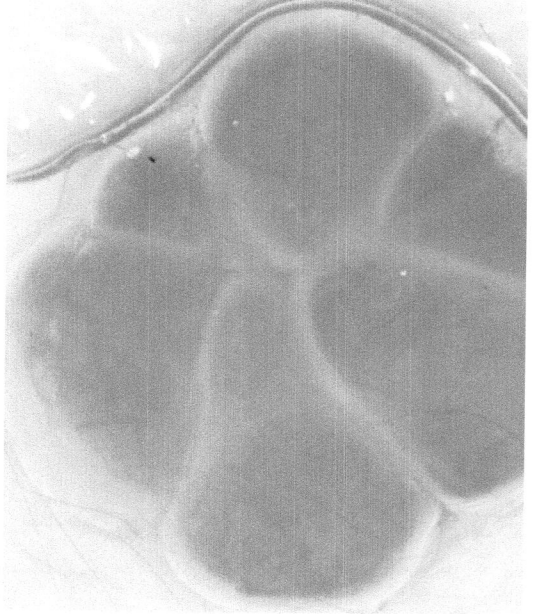

Fig. 1b

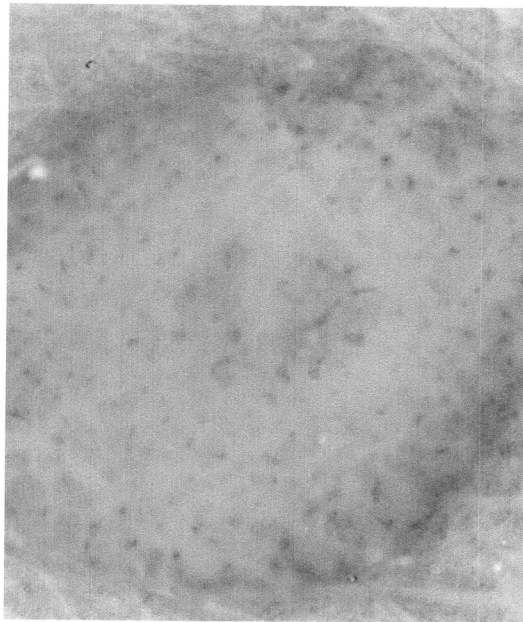

Fig. 2b

1. Hemangioma
2. Venous Malformation

Although their natural history is completely different, hemangioma and venous malformation may present with comparable clinical features, making the differential diagnosis difficult.

	1. Hemangioma	2. Venous Malformation
Definition	Benign tumor of vasoformative cells.	Malformation of venous vessels.
Frequency	4% of all pediatric skin disorders [5].	Less than 0.1% of all pediatric skin disorders [5].
Time of onset	Present at birth in 50% of cases.	Present at birth.
Initial clinical features	Usually, flat pink patch, sometimes ischemic with telangiectasias, livedoid. Rarely raised lesion.	Flesh-colored or red-bluish, compressible tumor, sometimes with coarse vessels.
Changes in the first few months	It grows, sometimes significantly.	It does not grow.
Changes in subsequent years	Slow, though significant, regression.	It becomes significantly more evident within decades.

Diagnostic Summary

Hemangioma: it grows in the first months of life and then regresses over a period of years.

Venous malformation: it does not grow in the first months and does not regress; rather, it progressively increases, though slowly, in size in decades.

1. Hemangioma

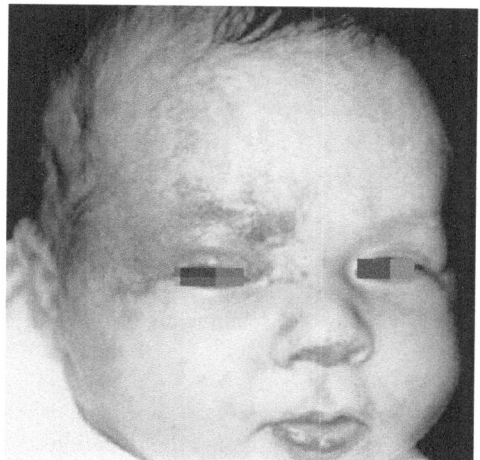

Fig. 1a

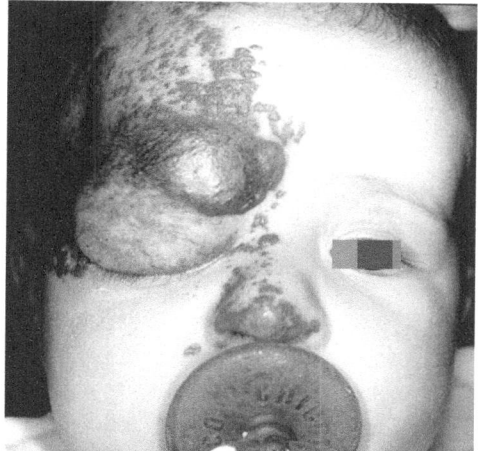

Fig. 1b Same patient as in Fig. 1a, aged 3 months

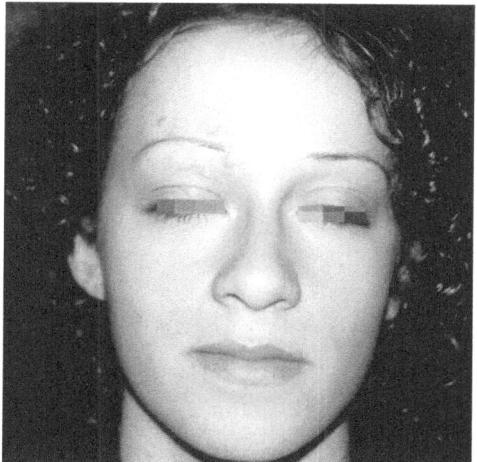

Fig. 1c Same patient as in Fig. 1a and 1b, aged 16 years

2. Venous Malformation

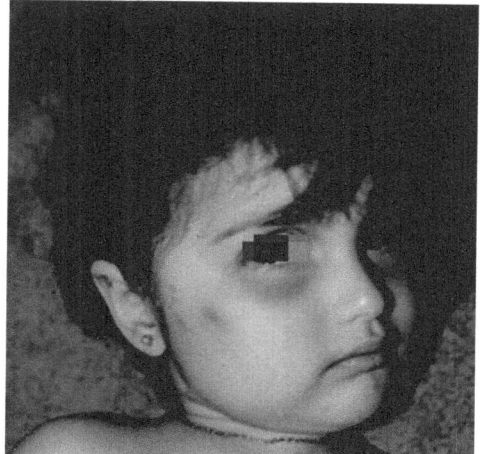

Fig. 2a

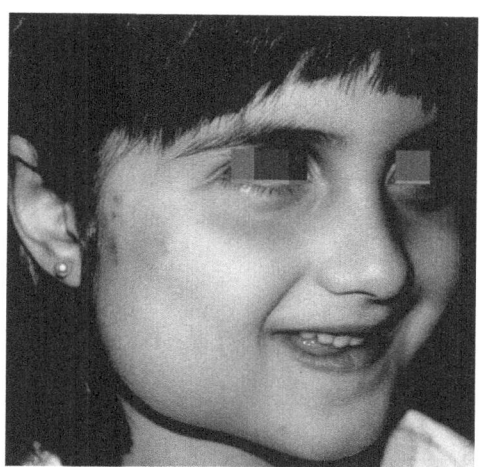

Fig. 2b Same patient as in Fig. 2a, aged 5 years

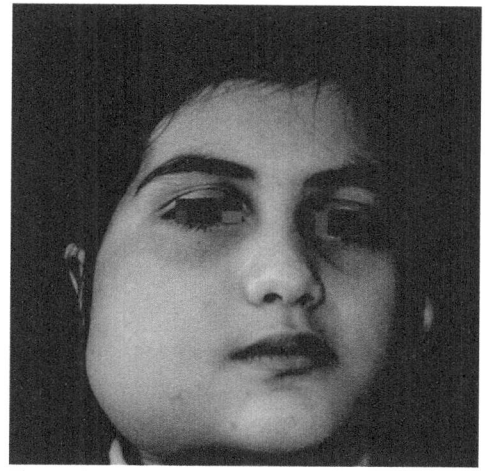

Fig. 2c Same patient as in Fig. 2a and 2b, aged 16 years

1. Nevus Anemicus
2. Ischemic Precursor of Hemangioma

Both nevus anemicus and ischemic precursor of hemangioma are characterized by cutaneous vasoconstriction, which makes differential diagnosis difficult.

	1. Nevus Anemicus	2. Ischemic Precursor of Hemangioma
Definition	Nevus due to persistent vasoconstriction of the papillary vessels.	Transient ischemic area followed by hemangioma.
Associated disorders	Neurofibromatosis [7], port-wine stain.	Hemangiomas at other locations, prematurity.
Affected sites	Usually the chest.	Everywhere, more often lower limbs.
Size	From a few centimeters to more than 10 cm in diameter.	1.5–6 cm in the localized forms; covering the entire limb in its metameric form.
Clinical features	White patch with polycyclic outline; often, at the periphery, white patches 1–2 mm in size, isolated, close together or partially confluent.	White patch with regular outline, usually roundish or segmental; often there are telangiectasias inside the ischemic patch.
Clinical course	It persists unchanged over time.	After hours or days, telangiectasias appear, followed by hemangioma which grows little and then regresses in months or years.

Diagnostic Summary

Nevus anemicus: patch with polycyclic outline remaining unchanged over time.

Ischemic precursor of hemangioma: roundish or metameric patch followed by hemangioma.

1. Nevus Anemicus

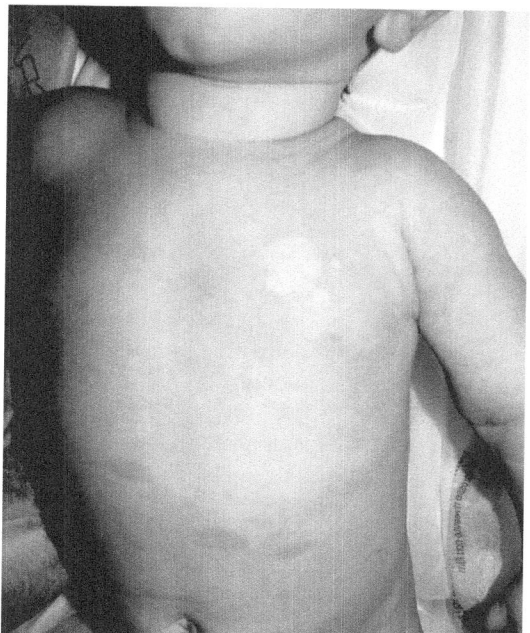

Fig. 1a Rubbing reddens only the surrounding skin

2. Ischemic Precursor of Hemangioma

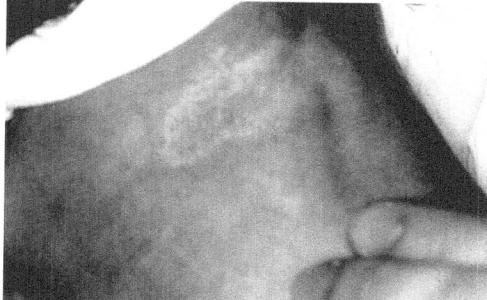

Fig. 2a At birth

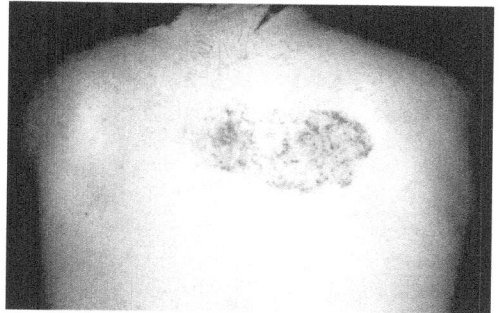

Fig. 2b Same child as in Fig. 2a, aged 3 months

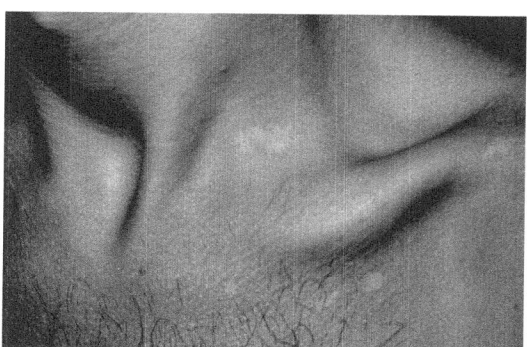

Fig. 1b An adult patient with nevus anemicus

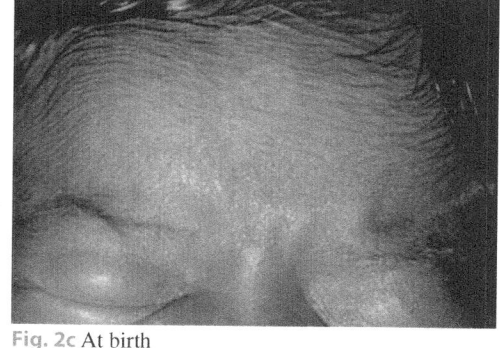

Fig. 2c At birth

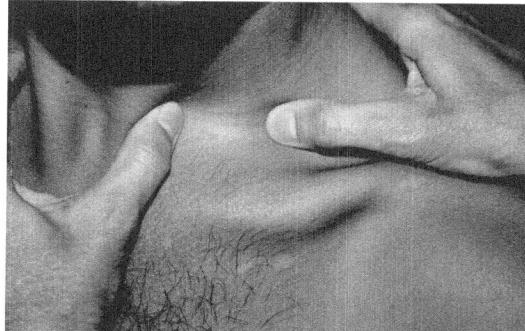

Fig. 1c Same patient as in Fig. 1b; under the pressure of the fingers the difference between nevus anemicus and the surrounding skin disappears

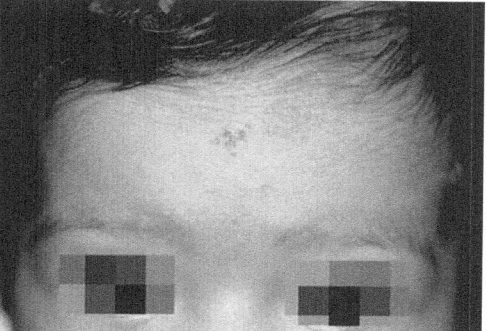

Fig. 2d Same child as in Fig. 2c, aged 3 months

1. Congenital Melanocytic Nevus
2. Hypermelanic Nevus

Some congenital melanocytic nevi are initially characterized by a generally uniform pale brown color (Fig. 1a). Therefore, they should be differentiated from hypermelanic nevi [8] devoid of cells (Fig. 2a).

	1. Congenital Melanocytic Nevus	2. Hypermelanic Nevus
Definition	Nevus consisting of melanocytes and/or nevus cells.	Nevus consisting of melanic pigment only.
Shape	Roundish, linear only in the palmar and plantar region.	Usually elongated.
Surface	Flat or palpable, sometimes with nodules.	Always flat.
Presence of terminal hairs	Frequent, especially after the first year.	Never.
Color	Usually blackish, sometimes light brown.	Always light brown, uniform.
Dermoscopy of light brown lesions	Sometimes hyperpigmented dots with melanocytic pattern (Fig. 1b).	Uniform hyperpigmentation (Fig. 2b).
Outline	Regular.	Often indented (Fig. 2a).
Clinical course	Changes in pigmentation, possible nodules, possible degeneration to melanoma.	Changes in pigmentation only with exposure to light. It cannot give rise to melanoma.

Diagnostic summary

Congenital melanocytic nevus: polymorphic, regular borders.

Hypermelanic nevus: monomorphic, indented borders.

1. Congenital Melanocytic Nevus

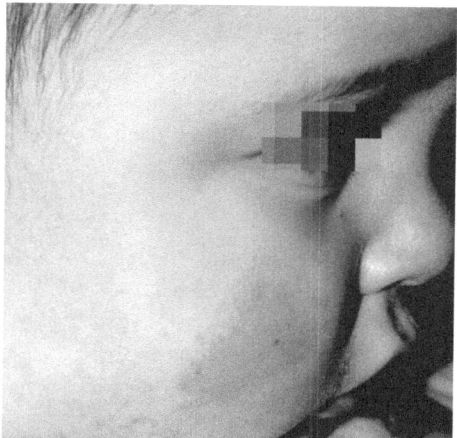

Fig. 1a Congenital melanocytic nevus
at the age of 3 months; two darker points stand
out on the hyperpigmented background

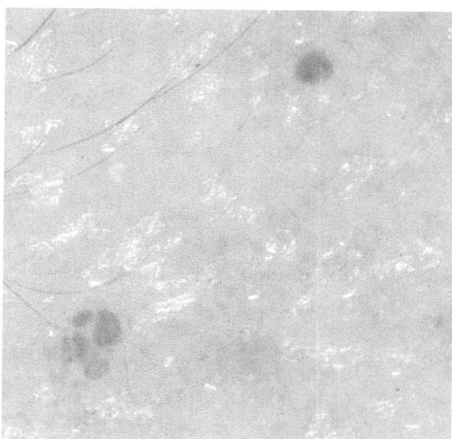

Fig. 1b Dermoscopy of Fig. 1a with
two hyperpigmented points

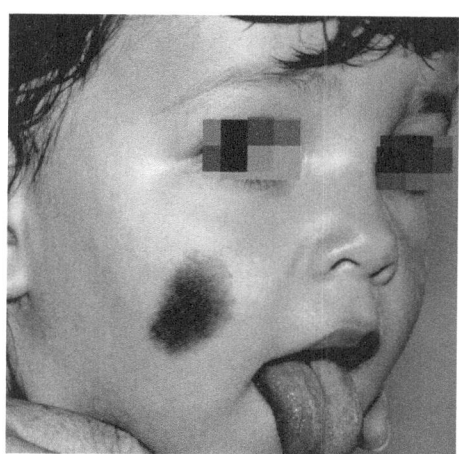

Fig. 1c The same child as in Fig. 1a at the age
of 1 year

2. Hypermelanic Nevus

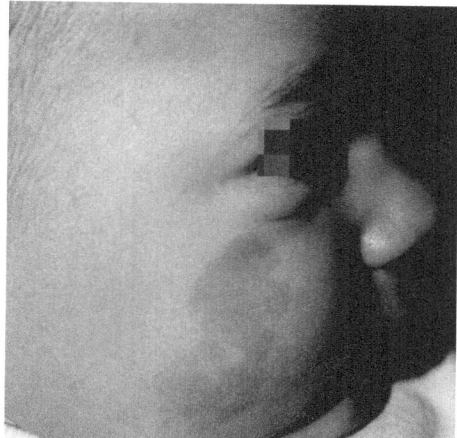

Fig. 2a Hypermelanic nevus at the age of
3 months; note the uniform hyperpigmentation
with indented borders

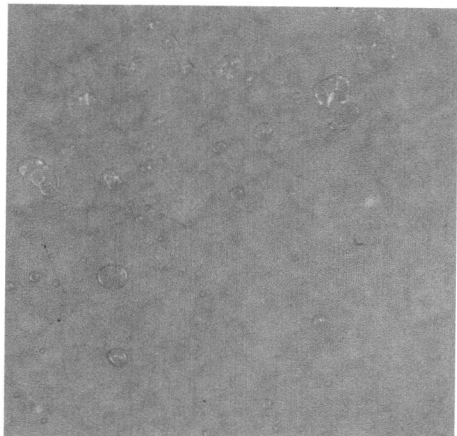

Fig. 2b Dermoscopy of Fig. 2a

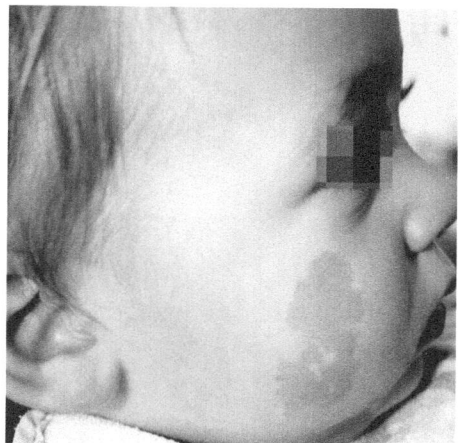

Fig. 2c The same child as in Fig. 2a at the age
of 1 year

1. Hypopigmented Spitz Nevus
2. Juvenile Xanthogranuloma

Hypopigmented Spitz nevus and juvenile xanthogranuloma are two generally rare, benign proliferations with a quite similar natural history. This is why they must be differentiated from each other, especially in the first month after onset, before xanthogranuloma becomes obviously yellow.

	1. Hypopigmented Spitz Nevus	2. Juvenile Xanthogranuloma
Definition	Benign proliferation of spindle and/or epithelioid melanocytes.	Benign proliferation of macrophage histiocytes.
Affected age	Incidence peak between 2 and 6 years.	Incidence peak in the first 2 years.
Dermoscopy	Dot-like vessels evenly distributed in the center of polygonal spaces identified by whitish septa (see Fig. 2a on page 15).	Pink-yellowish lesion, either amorphous or divided by whitish septa. Yellow image reminiscent of the setting sun, with peripheral erythema, telangiectasias, and sometimes a whitish network [9].
Color	Reddish (Fig. 1a).	Initially pink-brownish, then yellowish. After 1 month, yellow (Fig. 2a).
Clinical course	It grows for about 6 months and then tends to flatten out (Fig. 1b); undergoes regression with mild atrophy in about 2 years [6], or more rarely turns into a junctional or compound pigmented nevus.	After approximately 1 month, it turns yellow, grows for 3–6 months, then undergoes spontaneous regression (Fig. 2b) with mild atrophy in 2 years.

Diagnostic Summary

Hypopigmented Spitz nevus: on dermoscopy, it presents with regularly distributed dot-like vessels.

Juvenile xanthogranuloma: it becomes obviously yellow 1 month after onset.

1. Hypopigmented Spitz Nevus

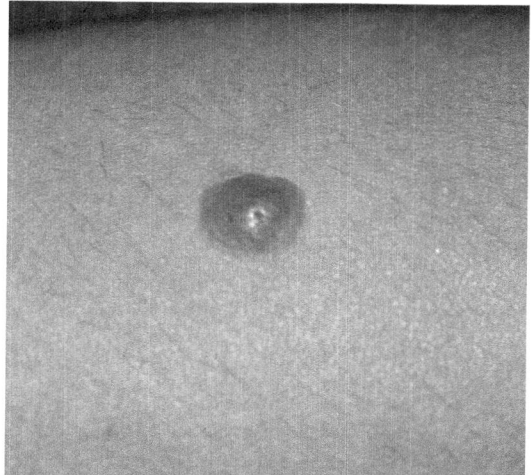

Fig. 1a

2. Juvenile Xanthogranuloma

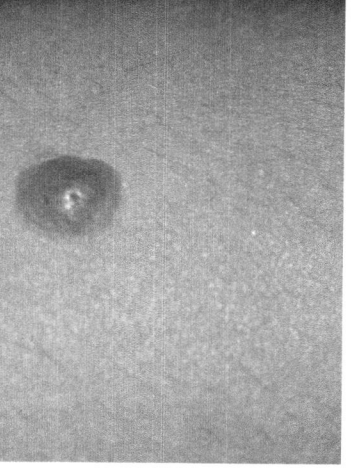

Fig. 2a

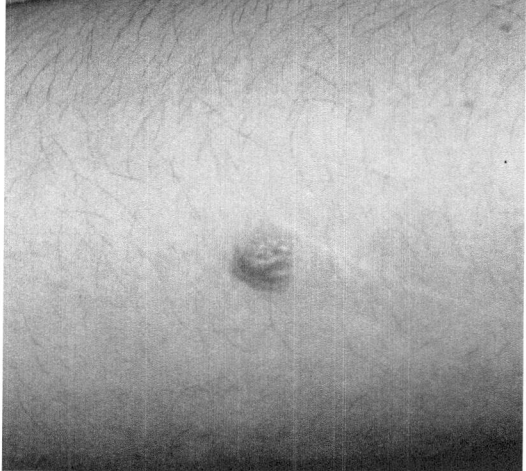

Fig. 1b Same child as in Fig. 1a after 2 years

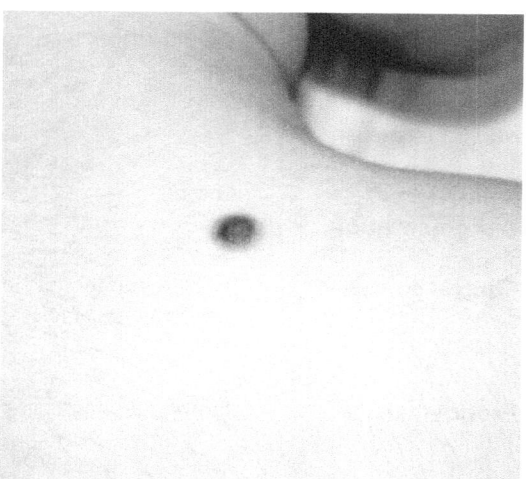

Fig. 2b Same child as in Fig. 2a after 2 years

1. Nevus Depigmentosus
2. Segmental Vitiligo

Nevus depigmentosus can affect a segment of skin with a distribution of lesions not unlike that of segmental vitiligo, hence the need for differential diagnosis between the two disorders.

	1. Nevus Depigmentosus	2. Segmental Vitiligo
Definition	Nevus malformation due to a defective transfer of melanin from the melanocyte to the keratinocyte.	Segmetal autoimmune disease due to a destruction of melanin.
Time of onset	Within the first year.	Usually, after the first year.
Lesion distribution	Single lesion (Fig. 1a), sometimes multiple lesions. The larger lesions tend to be distributed along the lines of Blaschko.	Single lesion, sometimes multiple lesions, but with segmental distribution; it may affect one half of the body.
Reddening on sun exposure	No.	Yes (Fig. 2a).
Follicular repigmentation	Absent.	Often present (Fig. 2b).
Clinical course	Persists throughout life without significant changes.	While persisting for many years, it undergoes significant changes and tends to improve significantly.
Prophylaxis	Photoprotection is not required.	Photoprotection of the lesions, and especially of the healthy surrounding skin, is required to prevent tanning, which makes the lesions more noticeable.

Diagnostic Summary

Nevus depigmentosus: remains unchanged over time, does not redden on sun exposure, and never presents follicular repigmentation.

Segmental vitiligo: it changes significantly and usually improves with time; reddens on exposure to the sun, and can present follicular repigmentation.

1. Nevus Depigmentosus

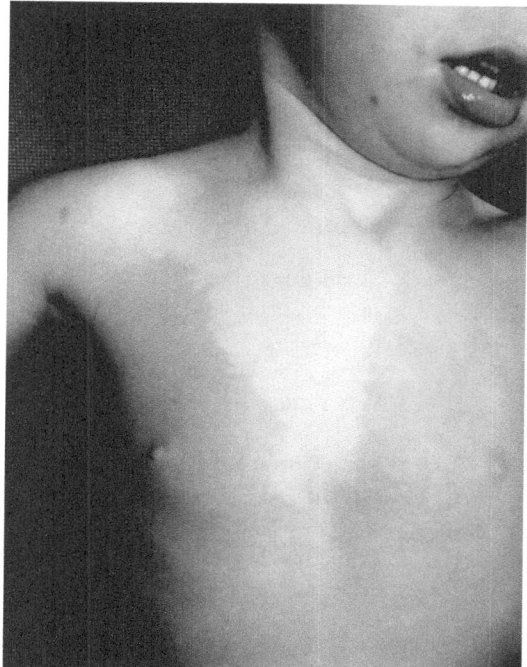

Fig. 1a

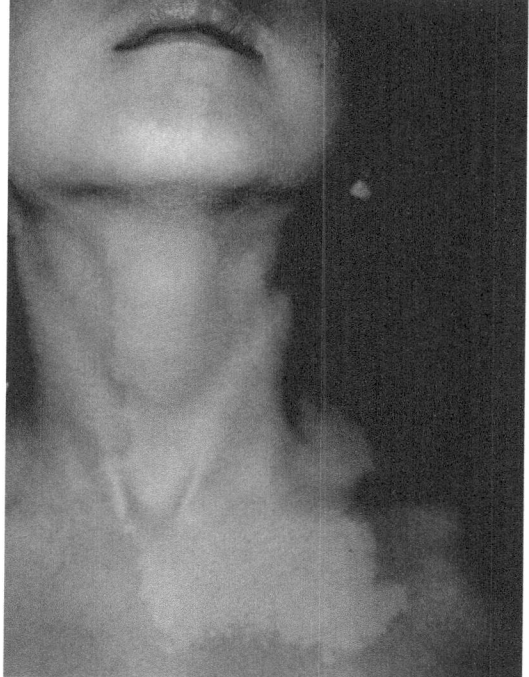

Fig. 1b

2. Segmental Vitiligo

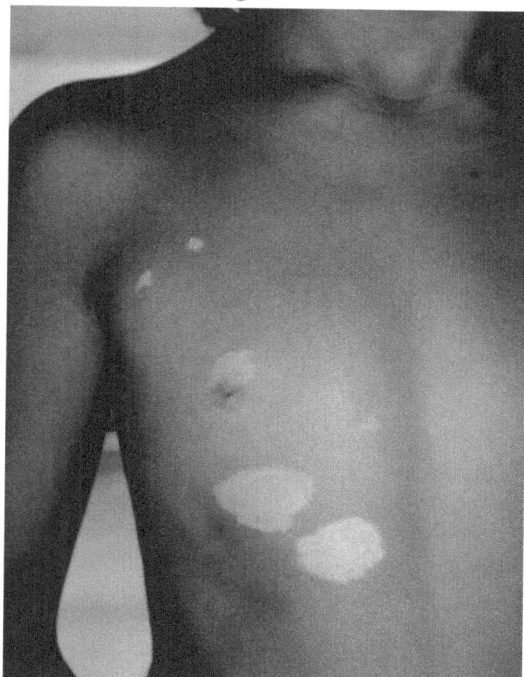

Fig. 2a Reddening of vitiligo on sun exposure

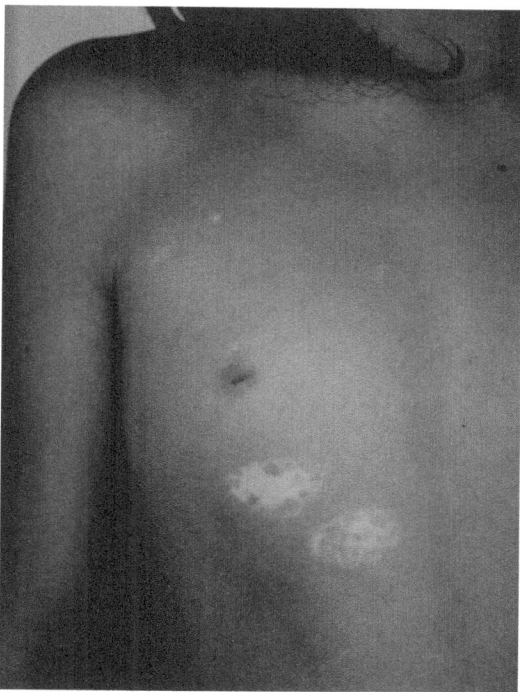

Fig. 2b Same child as in Fig. 2a, showing repigmentation

1. Nevus Depigmentosus
2. Nevus Anemicus

A single white spot on the skin at birth, or anyway in the early stages of life, is usually a nevus depigmentosus. However, nevus anemicus also manifests itself as a white spot from the earliest stages of life.

	1. Nevus Depigmentosus	2. Nevus Anemicus
Definition	Nevus due to abnormalities in the function of melanocytes.	Nevus due to persistent vasoconstriction of the papillary vessels.
Prevalence	0.4% of all dermatoses [5].	Very rare.
Associated disorders	Hyperpigmented nevus, hypomelanosis of Ito.	Neurofibromatosis, port-wine stain.
Clinical features	White patch with either indented or linear borders along the midline, sometimes linear distribution along the lines of Blaschko.	White patch. At its periphery, there are often 1–2 mm white areas, which are isolated, close to one another, or partially confluent.
Influence of the sun	After the first few years, clinical evidence of the nevus decreases with sun exposure.	Actinic erythema makes the nevus more evident, whereas tanning makes it less visible.
Diascopy of the periphery	The difference between healthy and hypopigmented skin does not change.	The peripheral healthy skin takes on the same color of the skin with nevus anemicus.
Rubbing	The hypopigmented skin reddens like the peripheral healthy skin.	The skin of nevus anemicus does not redden (Fig. 2b).

Diagnostic Summary

Nevus depigmentosus: frequent, under diascopy the difference with the peripheral healthy skin persists.

Nevus anemicus: rare; under diascopy, the difference between the nevus and healthy skin disappears; the skin of the nevus does not redden when rubbed.

1. Nevus Depigmentosus

2. Nevus Anemicus

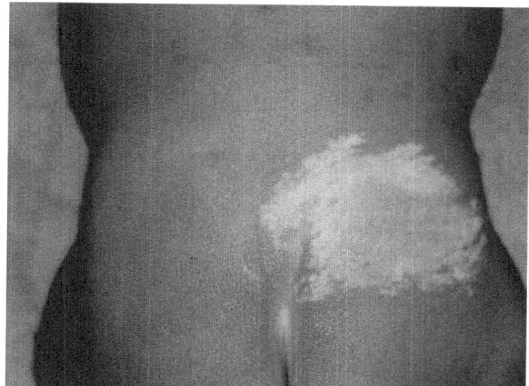

Fig. 1a

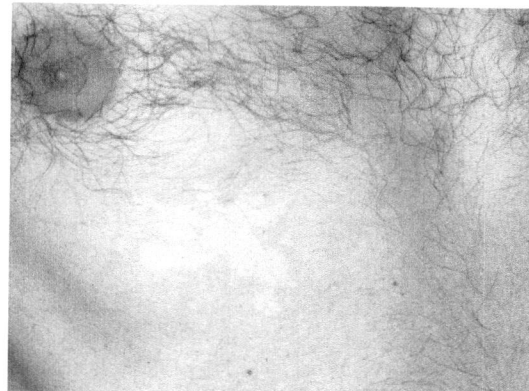

Fig. 2a

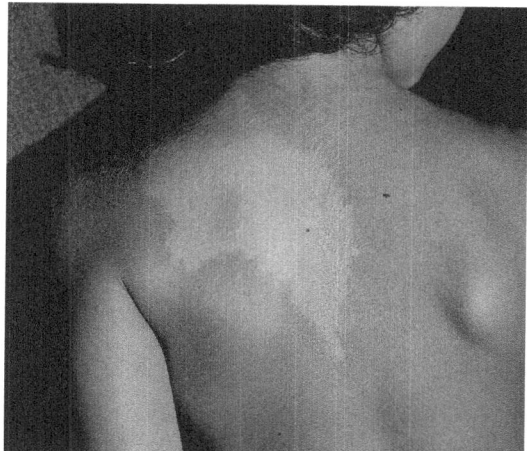

Fig. 1b

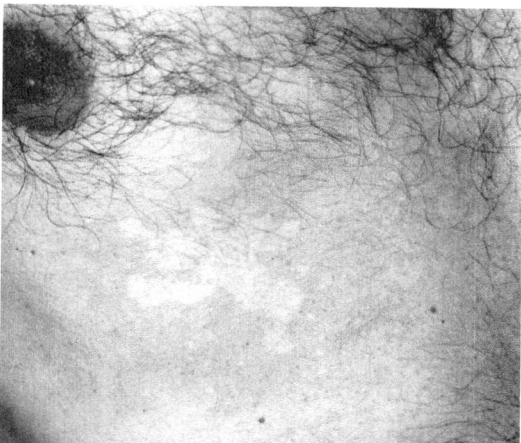

Fig. 2b Rubbing only redddens the peripheral, healthy skin

1. Epidermal Nevus
2. Lichen Striatus

Like most nevi, epidermal nevus is present at birth and persists indefinitely. Lichen striatus is an acquired disease, but like epidermal nevus is distributed segmentally along the lines of Blaschko [10], leading to the assumption that, in the affected segment, there exists a clone of mutated cells that are differently sensitive to a pathogenic virus (silent nevus).

	1. Epidermal Nevus	2. Lichen Striatus
Definition	Clonal proliferation of keratinocytes due to postzygotic mutation.	Dermatitis of the dermoepidermal junction on a silent nevus, possibly due to viruses[1].
Time of onset	Usually at birth.	First decade, usually after the first 2 years.
Initial lesions	Discolored, usually hyperpigmented.	Inflammatory, lichen-like papules, 1–3 mm in size.
Lesion persistence	Lifelong.	Regression after months or years, usually with hypopigmented sequelae; it does not recur.

Diagnostic Summary

Epidermal nevus: present at birth, remains in the same area of the body for life; lesions range from hyperpigmented to verrucous.

Lichen striatus: acquired disease, self-healing, with lesions ranging from lichen-like papules to hypopigmented sequelae.

---

[1]The segmental and mosaic distribution of lichen striatus along one or several Blaschko lines means that along these lines, a pre-existing clone of mutated cells can be present before the appearance of the disease. Their clinically silent mutation consists of a peculiar susceptibility to become affected by lichen striatus in the presence of its causative factors.

1. Epidermal Nevus

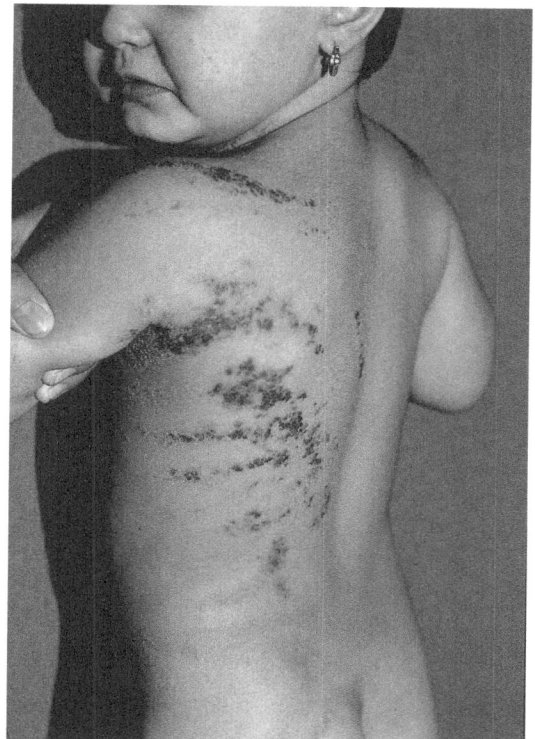

Fig. 1a

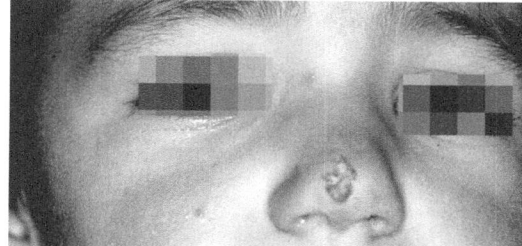

Fig. 1b

2. Lichen Striatus

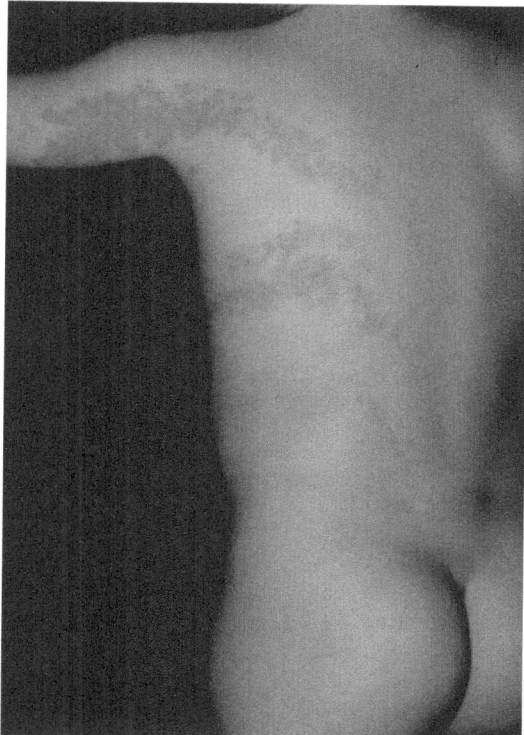

Fig. 2a

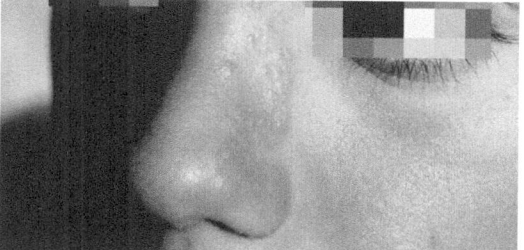

Fig. 2b

1. Verrucous Epidermal Nevus
2. Plane Warts

Verrucous epidermal nevus can be easily distinguished from plane warts thanks to its different history and for the different aggregation of its lesions. In some cases, however, epidermal nevus, especially in the palmar region, may not be apparent at birth and warts can, in turn, be distributed in a linear fashion, so as to require a differential diagnosis between the two diseases.

	1. Verrucous Epidermal Nevus	2. Plane Warts
Definition	Proliferation of keratinocytes induced by a mutation during fetal life.	Proliferation of keratinocytes induced by the human papillomavirus (HPV).
Time of onset	At birth or in the first years of life in the less widespread forms.	Usually after the second year of age.
Affected sites	Any cutaneous region.	Usually, the face and hands.
Surface	Initially flat, later on irregularly verrucous.	Flat.
Lesion distribution	Linear, along the lines of Blaschko.	Warts usually present on one side of the body. Linear lesions may be present as a result of trauma (Koebner phenomenon).
Lesion extent	1–50% of the cutaneous surface.	1–5% of the cutaneous surface.

Diagnostic Summary

Verrucous epidermal nevus: present at birth or from early on in life; it can be flat initially, but then becomes irregularly warty, and often follows a linear distribution.

Plane warts: appear after the second year of life, have a flat surface with little or no relief, tend to appear on one side of the body, where the initial center of infection can be often identified.

1. Verrucous Epidermal Nevus

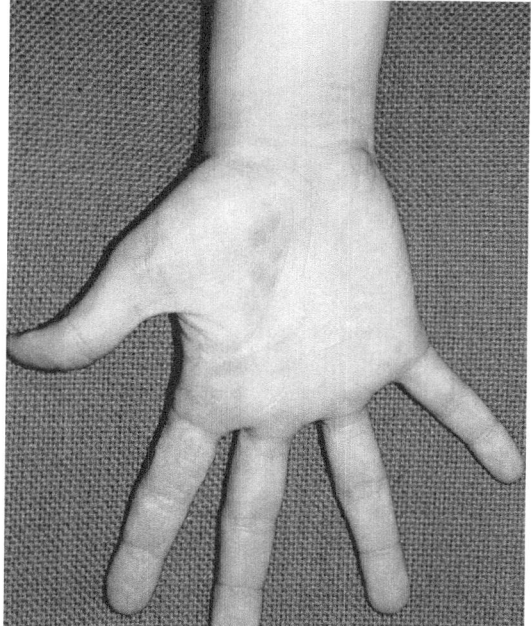

Fig. 1a

2. Plane Warts

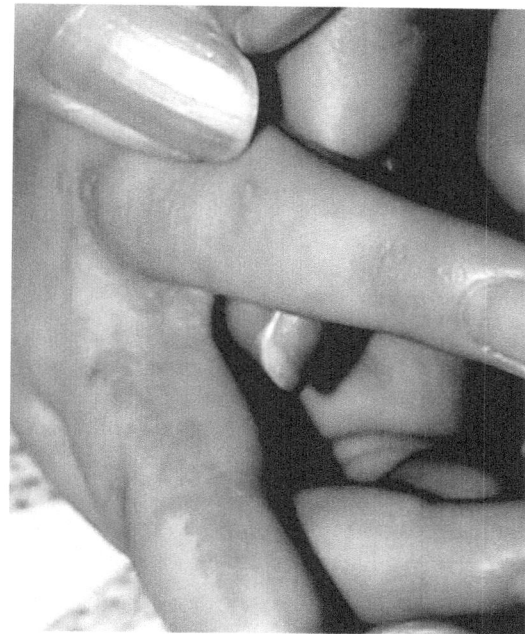

Fig. 2a

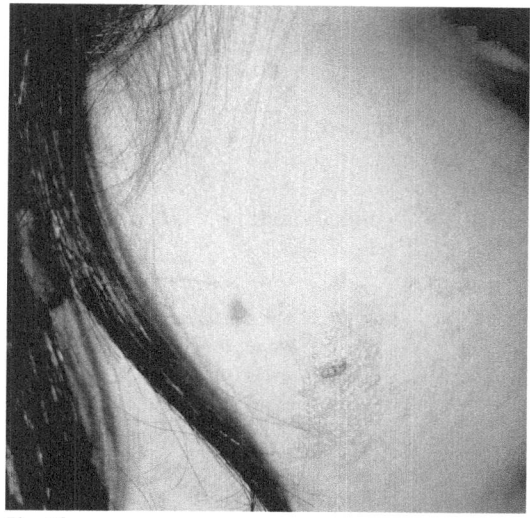

Fig. 1b

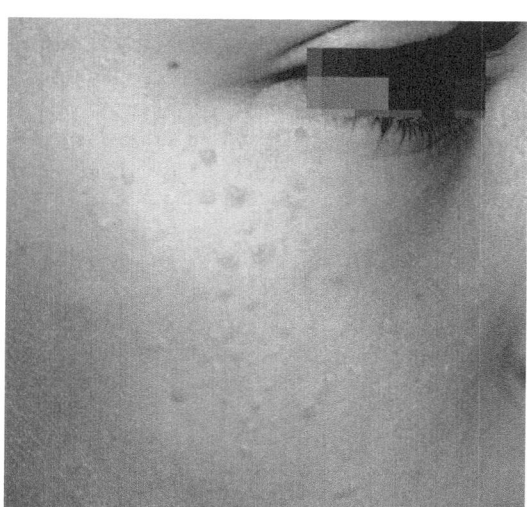

Fig. 2b

1. Sebaceous Nevus
2. Xanthogranuloma in Plaque of the Scalp

When a sebaceous nevus is roundish in shape, it can require a differential diagnosis from xanthomized juvenile xanthogranuloma in plaque of the scalp; in rare cases, a histological examination may become necessary.

	1. Sebaceous Nevus	2. Xanthogranuloma in Plaque of the Scalp
Definition	Localized hyperplasia of the epidermis, sebaceous glands, and sweat glands with hypotrophy of the hair.	Benign proliferation of dermal lipophage histiocytes; it undergoes progressive xanthomization before spontaneously regressing.
Time of onset	At birth.	It can occur at any age. It is present at birth in 9% of cases [11].
Number of lesions	One.	One in 62% of cases [11].
Lesion morphology	Roundish, oval, sometimes linear.	Roundish, sometimes irregular.
Relief	Just raised with respect to the surrounding skin.	Raised by a few millimeters.
Surface appearance	Granular or verrucous.	Smooth.
Color	White-yellowish, yellow suede.	Initially red-brownish, later on yellow.
Clinical course	Unchanged with time. Tumors, usually benign, can arise on the nevus [3].	It grows during the first months from its onset. Later on, it becomes progressively xanthomized and finally regresses within a couple of years.
Histological examination	Hyperplastic epidermis, hypertrophic sebaceous and sweat glands, hair is thin or absent.	Thinned epidermis; in the dermis, new formation of macrophages (lipophages) with Touton giant cells.

Diagnostic Summary

Sebaceous nevus: it is just raised off the skin surface, and has a granular or verrucous surface.

Xanthogranuloma in plaque of the scalp: initially reddish in color, it is raised by several millimeters and has a smooth surface.

Sebaceous Nevus vs. Xanthogranuloma in Plaque of the Scalp

33

1. Sebaceous Nevus

2. Xanthogranuloma in Plaque of the Scalp

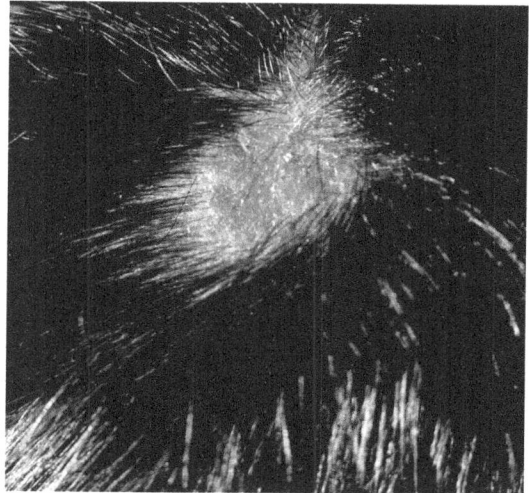

Fig. 1a

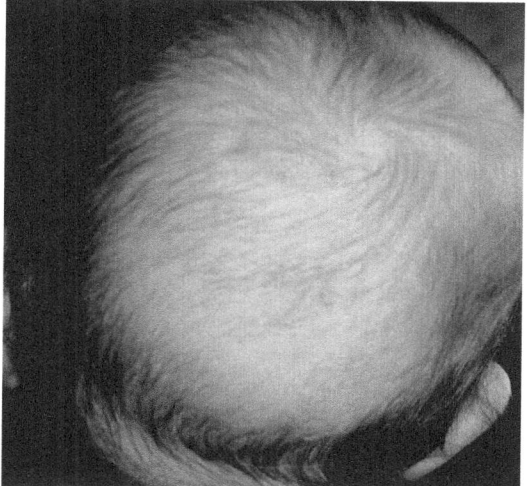

Fig. 2a

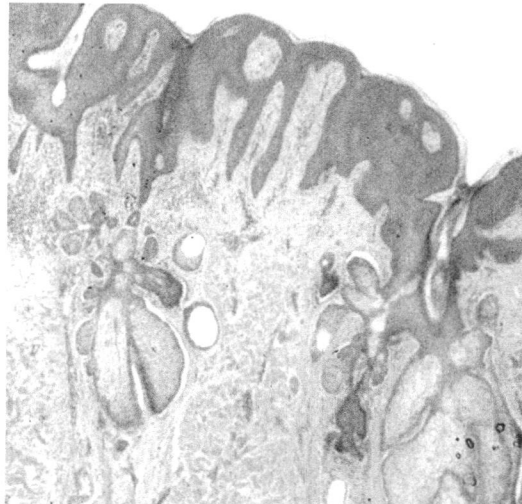

Fig. 1b

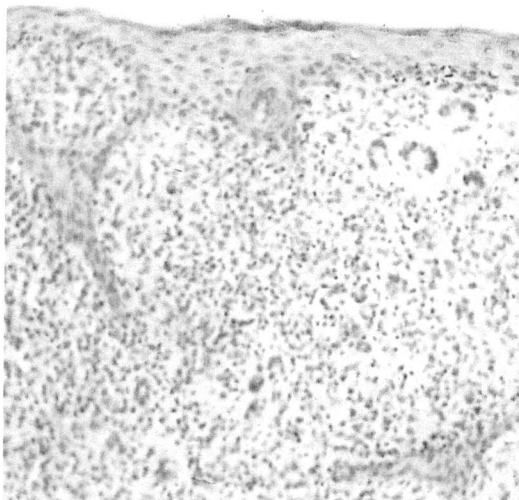

Fig. 2b

Nevi with Hypertrichosis

A localized hypertrichosis of the nevus type, i.e., due to a postzygotic mutation, occurs as an isolated phenomenon in nevus hypertrichosis, whereas it is associated to other proliferating skin components in congenital melanocytic nevus, Becker's nevus, and congenital smooth muscle hamartoma. Congenital melanocytic nevus is also important because, though rarely, it can degenerate into malignant melanoma. Moreover, physicians should remember that a localized nevus hypertrichosis of the midline can be the manifestation of a dermal sinus.

1. Congenital Melanocytic Nevus
2. Becker Nevus
3. Nevus Hypertrichosis
4. Congenital Smooth Muscle Hamartoma

	1. Congenital Melanocytic Nevus	2. Becker Nevus	3. Nevus Hyper-trichosis	4. Congenital Smooth Muscle Hamartoma
Definition	Nevus due to the proliferation of melanocytes.	Nevus due to increased sensitivity to androgens.	Nevus characterized by isolated hypertrichosis.	Nevus due to the proliferation of arrector pili muscle cells.
Difference between the sexes	No difference between the sexes.	It is more prevalent in males.	No difference between the sexes.	No difference between the sexes.
Time of onset of hypertrichosis	Usually 2–3 years, can be congenital.	Usually at puberty.	At birth.	At birth.
Nevus size	From a few millimeters to decimeters.	Usually, 10–12 cm.	Usually, 2–8 cm.	From 2 to 20 cm.
Color	Blackish.	Brown.	Skin-colored.	Skin-colored.
Palpation	Dermal infiltration is possible.	No obvious dermal infiltration.	No infiltration.	Transient hardening due to muscle contraction; occasionally, infiltrated plaque.
Clinical course	Regression/depigmentation in 7% of cases [12]. Otherwise, it persists indefinitely.	It tends to persist indefinitely.	It tends to persist indefinitely.	It tends to spontaneously regress within a matter of years.

1. Congenital Melanocytic Nevus

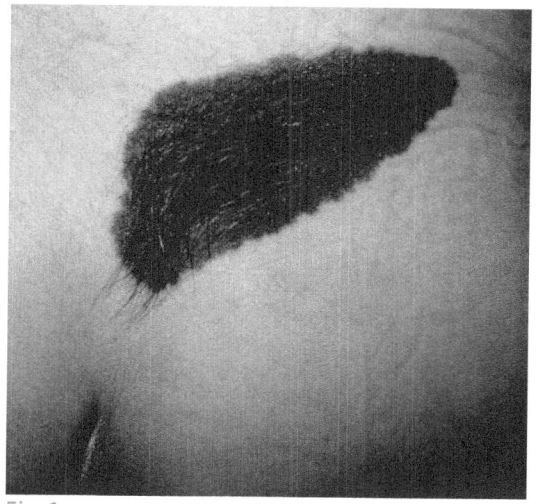

Fig. 1

2. Becker Nevus

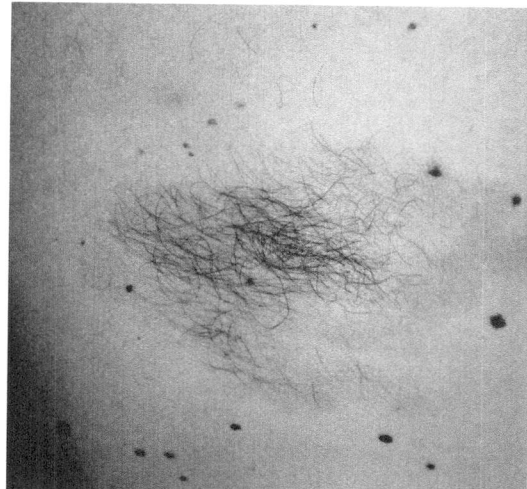

Fig. 2

3. Nevus Hypertrichosis

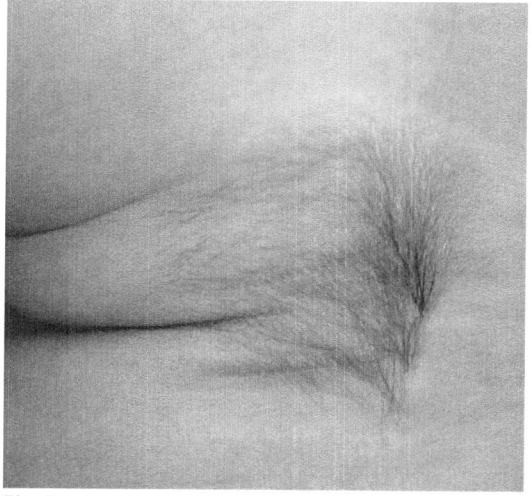

Fig. 3

4. Congenital Smooth Muscle Hamartoma

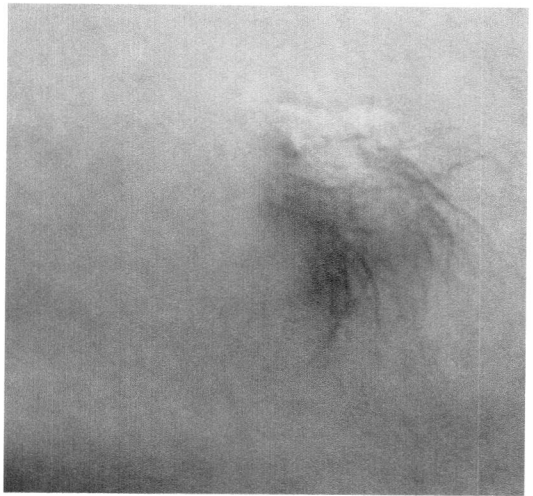

Fig. 4

Diagnostic Summary

Congenital melanocytic nevus: it is characterized by a blackish, often non-uniform, color.

Becker nevus: it appears or becomes more evident at puberty; it is uniformly brown in color.

Nevus hypertrichosis: skin-colored.

Congenital smooth muscle hamartoma: the lesion contracts when palpated.

Viral Infections

E. Bonifazi, *Differential Diagnosis in Pediatric Dermatology,*
DOI: 10.1007/978-88-470-2859-3_3 © Springer-Verlag Italia 2013

1. Herpes Zoster
2. Insect Stings with Zoster-Like Distribution

Both herpes zoster and insect stings start suddenly and are symptomatic. Some creeping insects can sting only a segment of the chest simulating herpes zoster.

	1. Herpes Zoster	2. Insect Stings with Zoster-Like Distribution
Environmental survey	Negative.	Exposure of the involved area to insects shortly before the onset of the lesions.
Pruritus	Present.	Present.
Burning pain	Present, but may be absent in young people; it has a metameric distribution.	Absent.
Lesion type	Reddish edematous lesions, rapidly becoming vesicles and then pustules.	Reddish papules, sometimes with central exudation. After a couple of days, the peripheral edema disappears and a small central papule persists.
Lesion distribution	Close lesions, often grouped in roundish areas, and regularly distributed in the involved dermatome.	Linearly or irregularly distributed lesions. Isolated lesions in other areas outside the interested metamere are frequently observed.
Regional adenopathy	Present; the regional lymph nodes are enlarged and tender.	Usually absent.
Clinical course	New vesicular lesions appear over several days; pustules become crusted over. Recovery is complete within 2–3 weeks when the crusts fall off.	Once contact with insects is eliminated, no new lesions occur and the eruption spontaneously regresses in a few days.

Diagnostic Summary

Herpes zoster: metameric burning paresthesias; the clearly exudative lesions are regularly distributed along one dermatome.

Insect stings with zoster-like distribution: they are itchy, have persistent papules, and have more irregular distribution.

1. Herpes Zoster

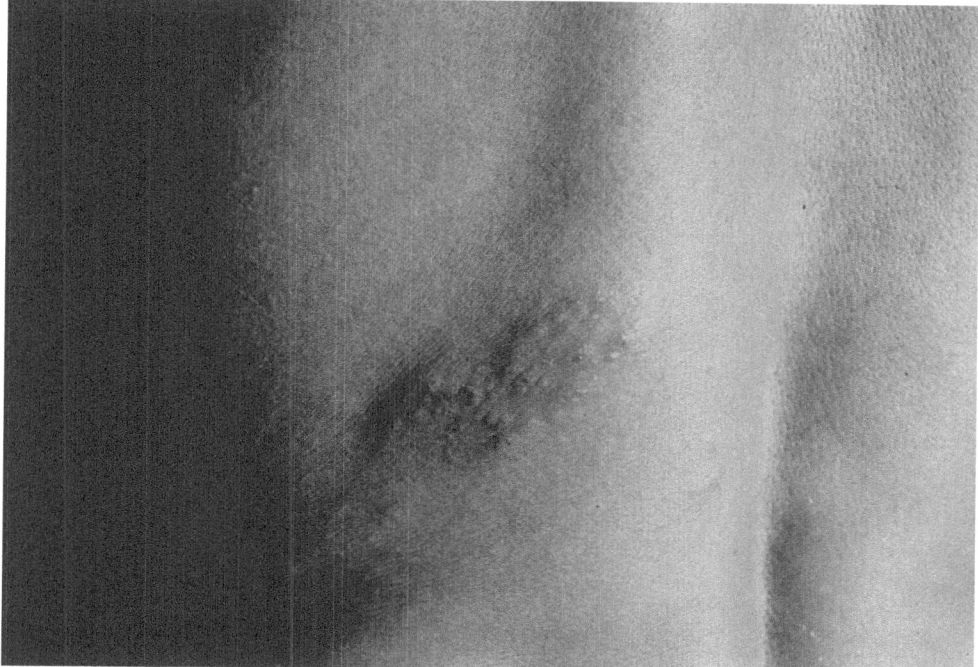

Fig. 1

2. Insect Stings with Zoster-Like Distribution

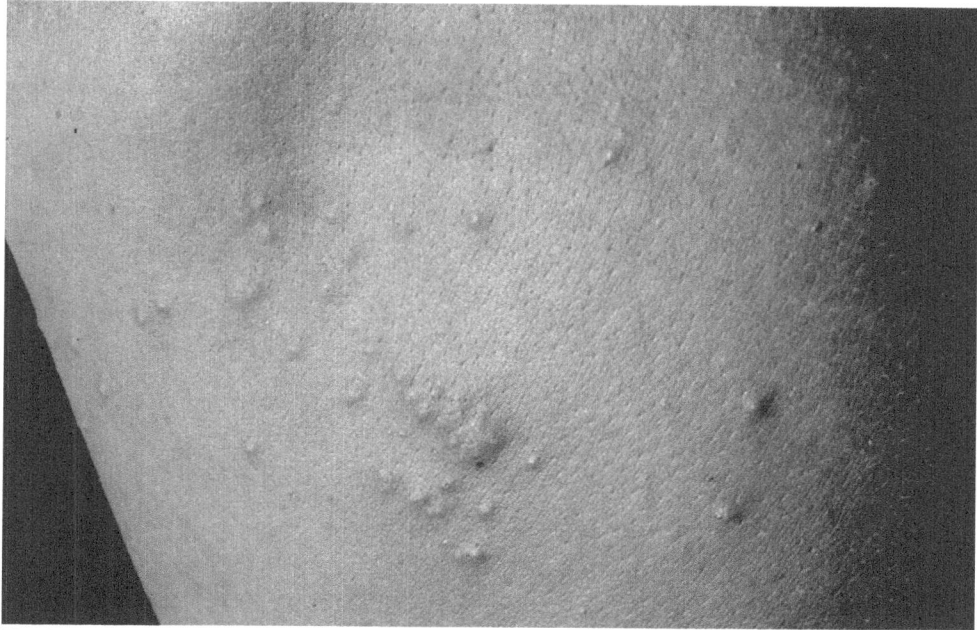

Fig. 2

1. Herpes Simplex
2. Pyoderma
3. Tinea

Crusted lesions on the face of a child may give rise to diagnostic doubt as to their etiology—herpes simplex virus, *staphylococcus aureus*, or fungi.

	1. Herpes Simplex	**2. Pyoderma**	**3. Tinea**
Etiology	Herpes simplex virus.	*Staphylococcus aureus.*	*Microsporum canis* (usually in Europe).
Seasonal frequency	Prevalent during winter and on first exposure to sunlight in summer.	Prevalent in hot and humid weather (mid-late summer).	Peaks twice a year, which is related to the birth of new kittens.
Contagiousness	Not evident, endogenous reinfection.	Evident, interpersonal.	Evident—interpersonal or from cat, dog, or rabbit.
Affected age	First decade.	First decade.	Any age.
Clinical features	Clustered pustules, erosions, and finally crusts.	Pustules and humid crusts of different sizes.	Erythematous and scaling lesions, more congested at the periphery, with central regression.
Pustules	Uniform, 1–2 mm in diameter.	Erode and progressively enlarge until they reach many centimeters.	Rare, 1–2 mm in size at the periphery.
Progression of lesions	They stay at the site where they occur on the first day.	They spread contiguously in days.	They spread contiguously in weeks.
Resolution	Spontaneous, within 7 days.	Due to antibiotics.	Due to antimycotics.
Recurrence	Common.	Rare.	Rare.

Diagnostic Summary

Herpes simplex: the first episode is characterized by clustered pustules of uniform diameter; recurrences at the same site are more easily diagnosed.

Pyoderma: pustules or blisters that break easily and continue to enlarge at the periphery in days; clear contagion by contiguity.

Tinea: erythematous and scaling lesions that enlarge at the periphery within weeks, regressing in the center; clear contagion by contiguity.

1. Herpes Simplex

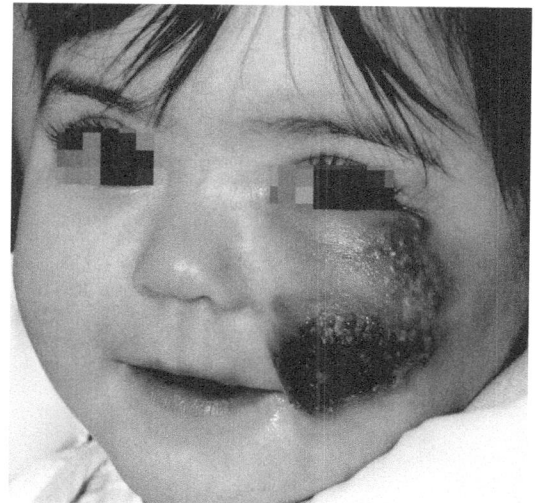

Fig. 1

2. Pyoderma

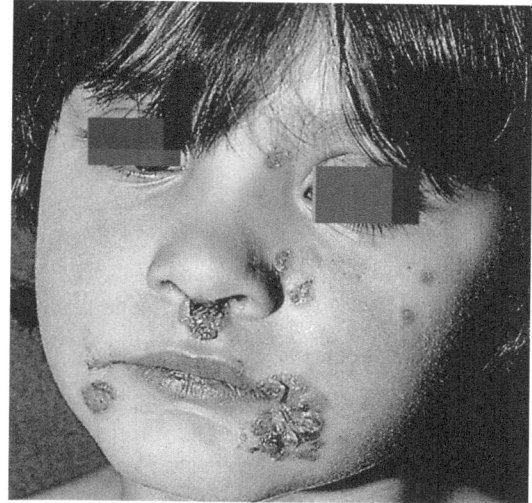

Fig. 2

3. Tinea

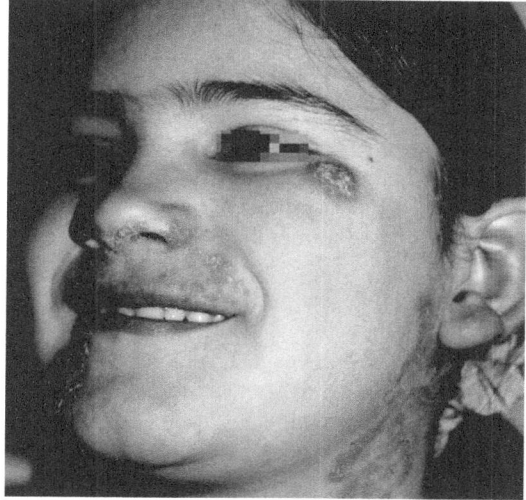

Fig. 3

1. Plane Warts
2. Benign Cephalic Histiocytosis

Plane warts and benign cephalic histiocytosis affect mainly the face; morphologically, their lesions may also create problems of differential diagnosis.

	1. Plane Warts	**2. Benign Cephalic Histiocytosis**
Definition	Papules due to keratinocyte proliferation induced by human papillomavirus (HPV).	Papules due to benign proliferation of histiocytes.
Prevalence	Very frequent: 1.4% of all pediatric skin disorders [5].	Very rare.
Time of onset	Usually, after the second year of life.	First 2 years of life.
Lesion distribution	Usually asymmetrical. The lesions are more numerous at the first side to be affected.	Symmetrical on both cheeks.
Lesion location	Face, dorsal surface of the hand.	Face, sometimes the upper chest.
Lesion type	Flat papules, 1–4 mm in diameter.	Flat or hemispheric papules, 2–3 mm in diameter.
Clinical course	The lesions spontaneously regress without sequelae after months or years. Their regression often occurs suddenly.	The lesions regress spontaneously, but slowly, over a period of 2–5 years. The larger lesions sometimes leave a slight atrophy or a pigmented macula.

Diagnostic Summary

Plane warts: are distributed asymmetrically, and are more numerous at the initial center of infection; they appear after the second year.

Benign cephalic histiocytosis: randomly distributed bilaterally on the face; begins in the first two years of life.

1. Plane Warts

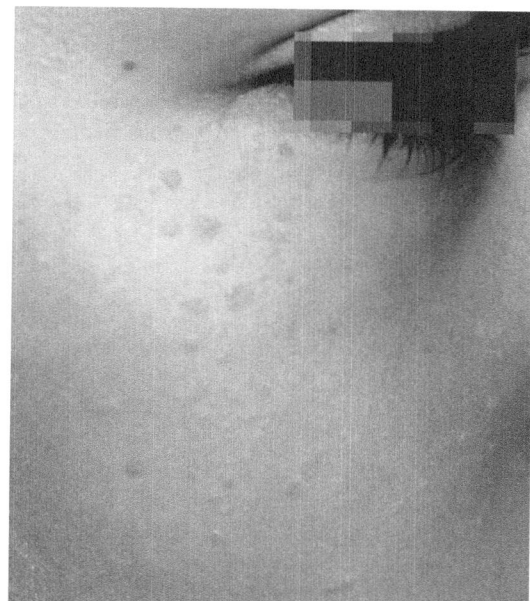

Fig. 1

2. Benign Cephalic Histiocytosis

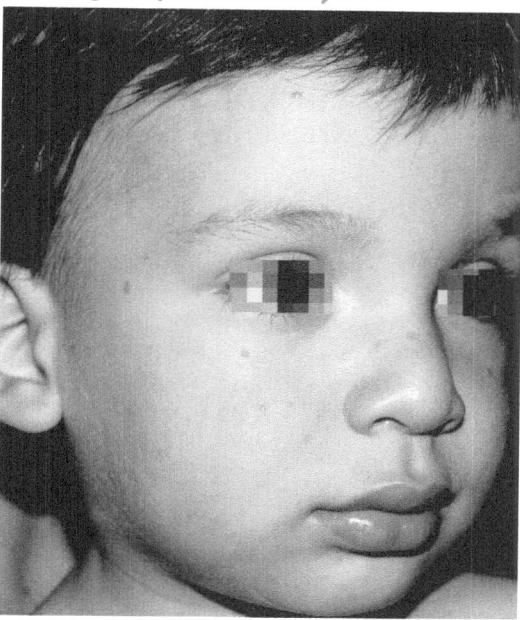

Fig. 2

1. Vulvar Epidermal Nevus
2. Genital Warts

Genital warts can affect the vulvar region; they often have an early onset, even appearing in the first months of life, and persist for a long time, sometimes requiring differential diagnosis from an epidermal nevus.

	1. Vulvar Epidermal Nevus	2. Genital Warts
Definition	Clonal proliferation of keratinocytes, secondary to fetal mutation.	Epidermal neoplasms induced by HPV.
Pathogenesis	Secondary to a mutation.	Follows a perinatal infection from relatives with cutaneous or genital warts, or rarely due to abuse; it is usually innocent in the first 3 years of life.
Lesion onset	At birth or in the first months of life.	After the first few weeks of life, even in the case of perinatal infection.
Primary skin lesions	Maculae, flat or verrucous papules.	Thread-like, flat, or verrucous papules.
Lesion location	Unilateral, usually linear.	Usually bilateral.
Lesion surface	Initially flat, becoming raised with time.	Raised from the outset.
Clinical course	Initially flat or only just raised, it tends to thicken irregularly over time and does not regress.	They tend to persist for years, but changing in number; when removed, they tend to reappear for years. In the end, they regress spontaneously.

Diagnostic Summary

Vulvar epidermal nevus: usually unilateral and linear; its initially flat lesions thicken with time; it never regresses.
Genital warts: usually bilateral, their lesions vary in number with time and eventually spontaneously regress.

1. Vulvar Epidermal Nevus

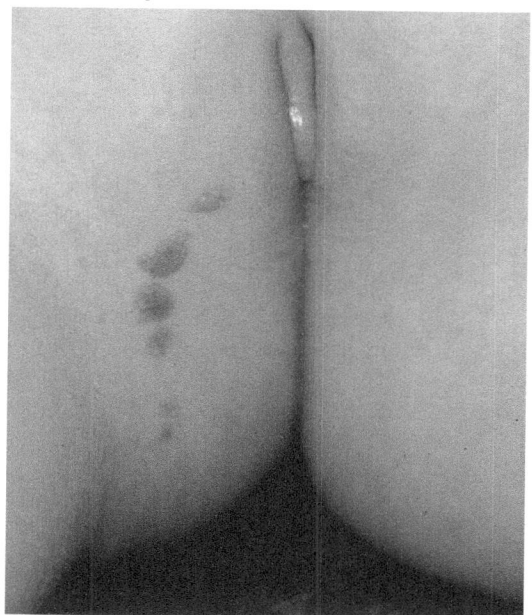

Fig. 1a

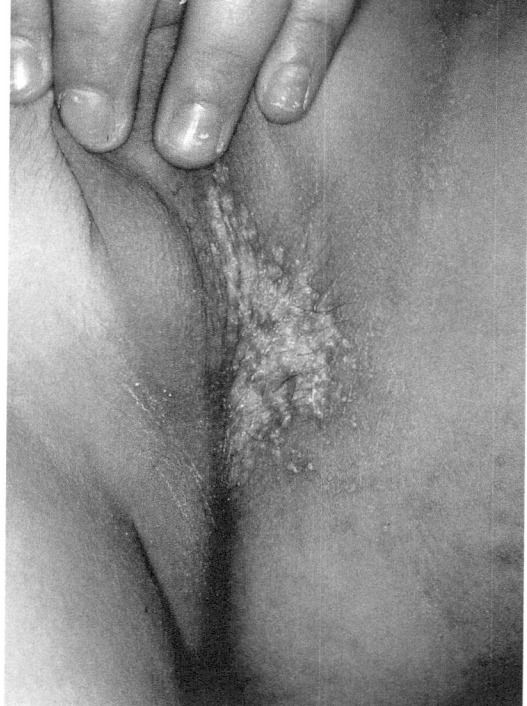

Fig. 1b

2. Genital Warts

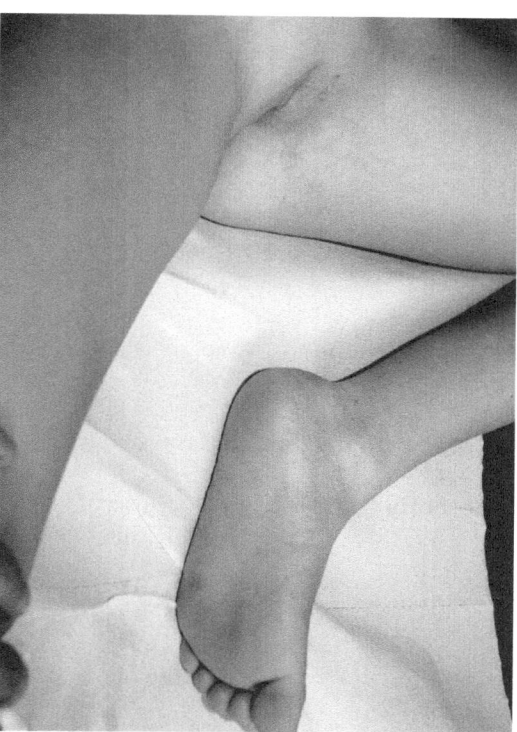

Fig. 2a

Fig. 2b The same child as in Fig. 2a; beside genital warts, plantar wart is also visible

1. Common Warts
2. Subungual Exostosis

When they involve the subungual region, common warts and exostosis can present similar clinical features giving rise to diagnostic doubts.

	1. Common Warts	**2. Subungual Exostosis**
Definition	Proliferation of keratinocytes caused by HPV.	Hamartoma caused by the proliferation of subperiosteal metaphyseal cartilage.
Prevalence	Frequent.	Rare.
Time of onset	First decades, after the third year of life.	First decade, between 6 and 10 years.
Difference between the sexes	No difference between the sexes.	More frequent in males.
Most prevalent location	Fingers and plantar aspect of foot.	Big toe, at the dorsomedial site.
Size	2–10 mm.	5–6 mm.
Surface	Verrucous.	Smooth, sometimes scaling.
Color	Grayish, blackish.	Pink.
Other lesions	History or finding of other warts nearby.	Absence of other lesions.
Relation with the bone	Superficial, movable on the deeper layer.	Adherent to the underlying bone.
Relation with the nail	Occasional onycholysis.	Frequent onycholysis.
Laboratory tests	Koilocytosis of keratinocytes on histological examination (Fig. 1b).	On X-ray examination, proliferation of bone tissue adherent to the underlying bone (Fig. 2b).

Diagnostic Summary

Common warts: verrucous surface, do not adhere to the deep layer.
Subungual exostosis: covered by healthy, smooth skin, adheres to the underlying bone.

1. Common Warts

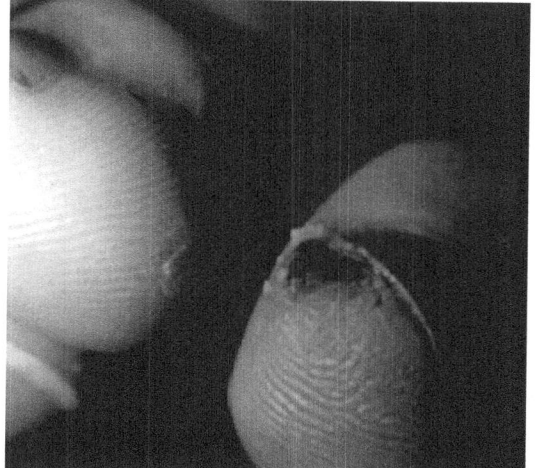

Fig. 1a

2. Subungual Exostosis

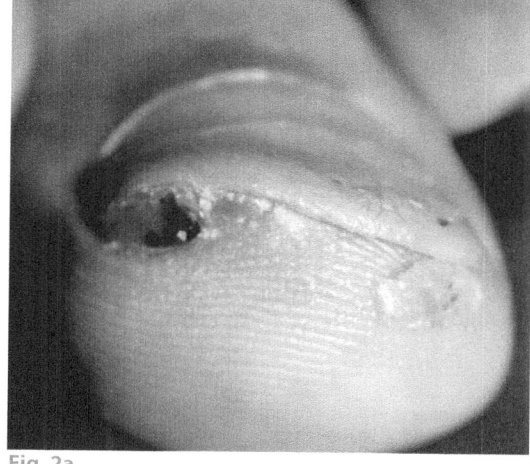

Fig. 2a

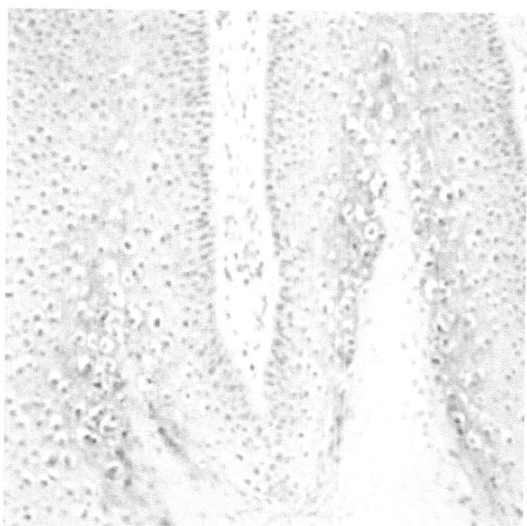

Fig. 1b Koilocytosis of the common warts

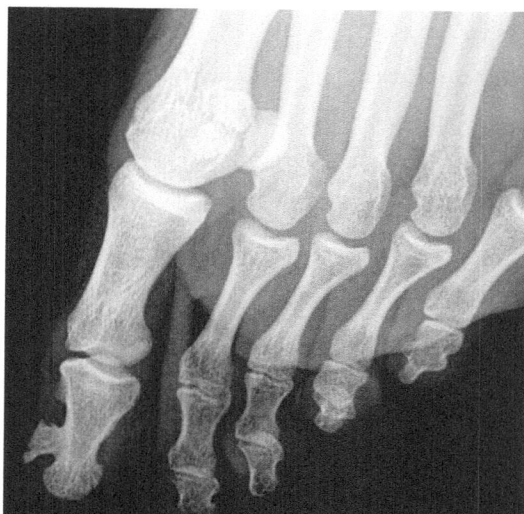

Fig. 2b X-ray evidence of exostosis

1. Perianal Condylomata Acuminata
2. Condylomata Lata of Congenital Syphilis

Besides the name, these two disorders share only the involved site, namely the perianal region; this is the classic location of condylomata lata of congenital syphilis and, in children, also the most frequent location of condylomata acuminata.

	1. Perianal Condylomata Acuminata	2. Condylomata Lata of Congenital Syphilis
Definition	Epidermal neoplasms caused by HPV.	Inflammatory dermal papules, due to recent congenital syphilis.
Prevalence	They represent 0.28% of all pediatric skin disorders [5]. In the first 12 years of life, the perianal location of these warts is by far the most frequent.	Congenital syphilis is rarer today, due to the fear of AIDS [14].
Pathogenesis	The pathogenesis of perianal and genital warts in the first few years of life is exceptionally linked to sexual abuse, unlike what happens in the peripubertal period. Often, no-one in the family of the patient has genital warts; occasionally, a relative may suffer from common warts of the hands.	Congenital syphilis is acquired by the fetus after the fourth month of pregnancy due to transplacental transmission. Condylomata lata correspond to a secondary papular syphiloderma and are significant of recent syphilis. They are related to the hematogenous dissemination of *Treponema pallidum*.
Lesion shape	Multiple neoplasms with greater axis perpendicular to the skin surface. Confluent lesions have a "cauliflower" appearance.	Inflammatory papules or plaques with a tendency to assume a circinate appearance.
Clinical course	They tend to persist for years and, when removed, they tend to recur for years. In the end, they regress spontaneously.	They regress permanently in weeks following specific treatment with penicillin.

Diagnostic Summary

Perianal condylomata acuminata: relief with greater axis perpendicular to the skin surface, occasionally flat.
Condylomata lata of congenital syphilis: inflammatory, circinate papules or plaques.

1. Perianal Condylomata Acuminata

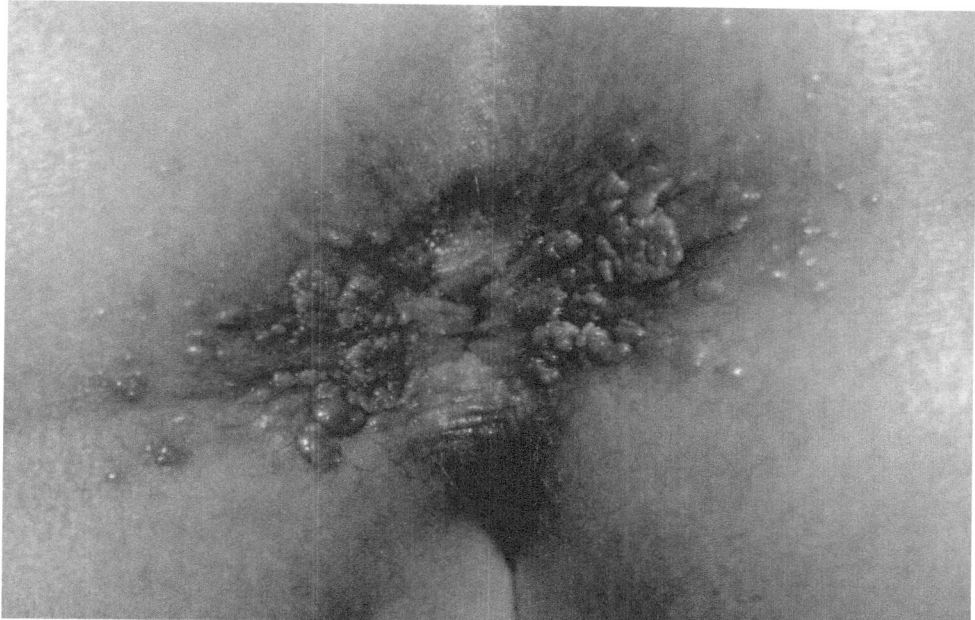

Fig. 1

2. Condylomata Lata of Congenital Syphilis

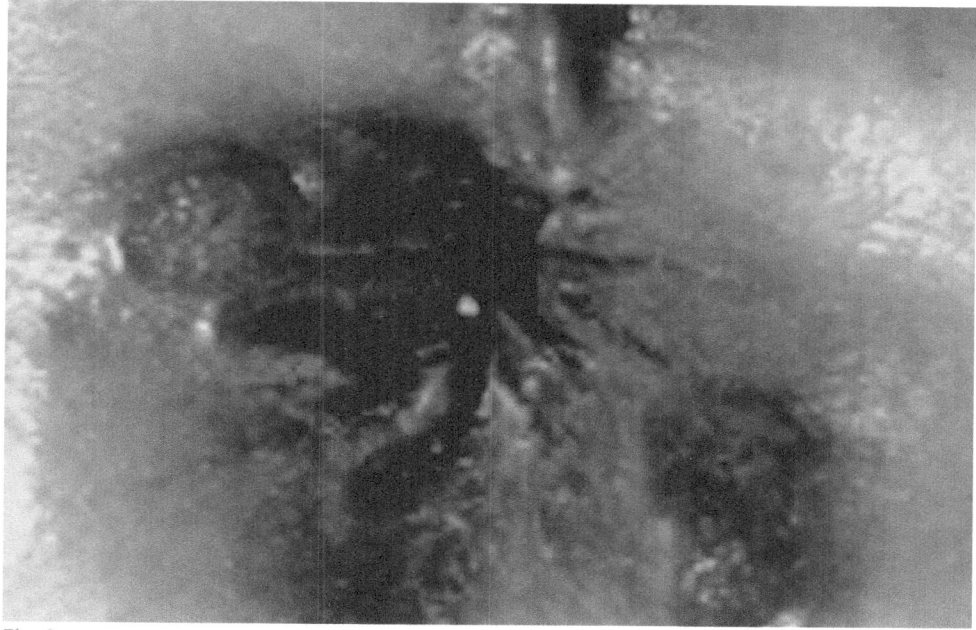

Fig. 2

1. Genital Warts
2. Pearly Penile Papules

Genital warts in children must be differentiated from a different physiological condition, the so-called pearly penile papules. This physiological condition is manifest in the peripubertal period and is responsible for major psychological problems when the adolescent is particularly sensitive to problems affecting the genital area.

	1. Genital Warts	2. Pearly Penile Papules
Cause	HPV.	Physiological condition.
Time of onset	Any age starting from the first few months of life.	Peripubertal.
Lesion location	Perianal, perigenital.	Basis of the glans penis.
Skin involvement	Possible.	Never.
Number of lesions	Variable; from one to dozens.	Dozens.
Lesion size	Variable; from 1 mm to several centimeters.	Uniform; 1 mm wide, 1–2 mm long.
Lesion confluence	Frequent.	Never.
Lesion shape	Cockscomb-like papules, cauliflower-like in the case of confluence.	Thread-like papules.
Clinical course of lesions	They persist for years, recurring regardless of the treatment used to remove them; eventually they disappear spontaneously.	Once noticeable, they persist with time, although their clinical evidence significantly changes with time.

Diagnostic Summary

Genital warts: they can appear at any age in the perianal and/or perigenital area.
Pearly penile papules: they become noticeable in the peripubertal period at the basis of the penile gland; they never appear on the skin and are regularly distributed.

1. Genital Warts

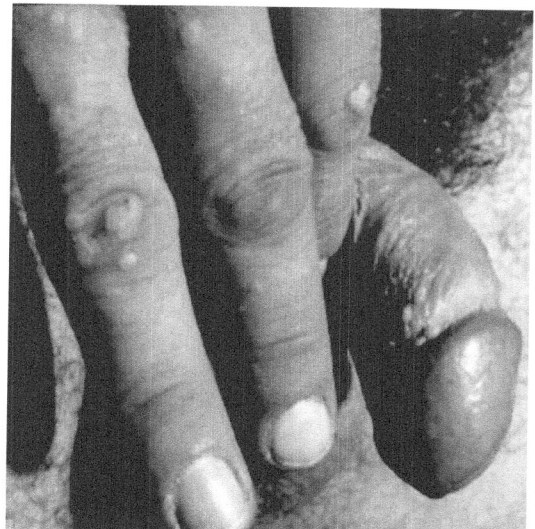

Fig. 1

2. Pearly Penile Papules

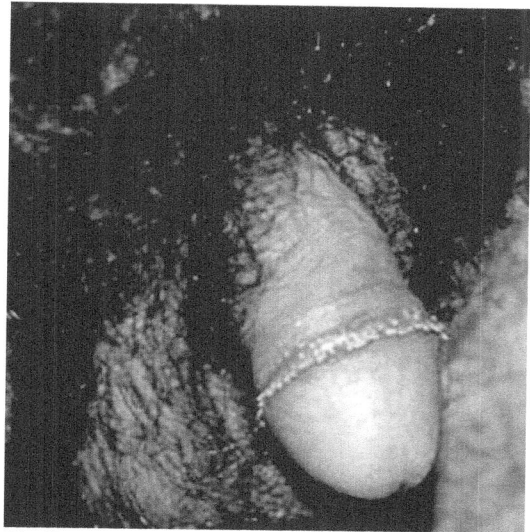

Fig. 2

1. Perianal Condylomata Acuminata
2. Infantile Perianal Protrusion

Condylomata acuminata in children almost always affect the perianal area. The latter is also the location of infantile perianal protrusion, which can be problematic when diagnosing each condition.

	1. Perianal Condylomata Acuminata	2. Infantile Perianal Protrusion
Definition	Localized epidermal proliferation caused by HPV, usually type 6 or 11.	Perianal skin protrusion of various etiology, congenital, associated to lichen sclerosus, constipation, diarrhea, and perianal dermatitis. Often, no cause can be demonstrated [15].
Difference between the sexes	No difference between the sexes.	It is prevalent in females.
Site	Perianal, perigenital, inguinal.	Anterior, or more rarely, the posterior perianal region.
Number of lesions	Numerous, often dozens.	One, rarely two.
Lesion shape	Thread-like or flat papules, sometimes confluent, forming cauliflower-like plaques.	Papule or flat nodule reminiscent of a pen shell (*Pinna nobilis*).
Lesion size	1–3 mm.	From a few millimeters to 1 cm.
Lesion color	Pink, whitish, brownish.	Pink.
Lesion surface	Irregular, cockscomb- or cauliflower-like.	Smooth.
Clinical course	They often recur regardless of the type of treatment; eventually, after several years, they disappear spontaneously.	Generally, it persists indefinitely.

Diagnostic Summary

Perianal condylomata acuminata: multiple lesions; their number changes (increases/decreases) significantly over time.
Infantile perianal protrusion: single lesion; it usually persists unchanged over time.

1. Perianal Condylomata Acuminata

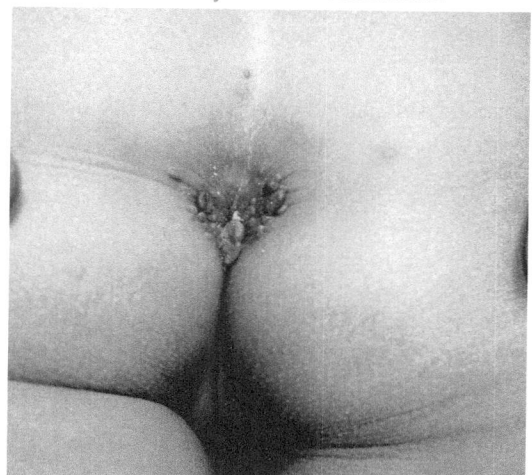

Fig. 1

2. Infantile Perianal Protrusion

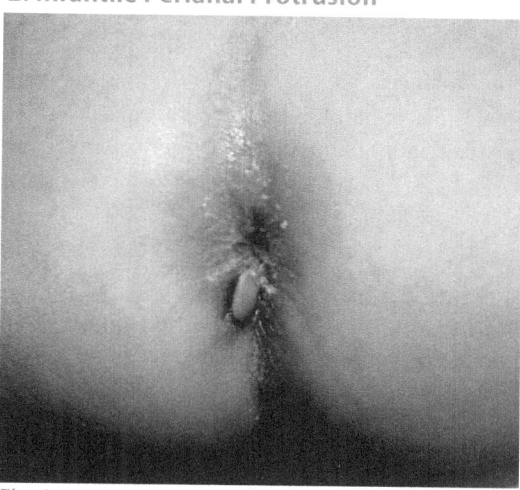

Fig. 2

1. Molluscum Contagiosum
2. Genital Warts

The lesions of molluscum contagiosum can be localized to the perianal and perigenital area in children, making the differential diagnosis with genital warts problematic.

	1. Molluscum Contagiosum	2. Genital Warts
Definition	Localized epidermal hyperplasia caused by a member of the poxvirus family.	Localized epidermal hyperplasia caused by HPV.
Age affected	From the first year of life through to adolescence.	From the first year of life to adulthood.
Clinical features	Translucent papules, with the larger lesions sometimes having a small central depression.	Whitish papules, often with an irregular surface.
Lesion size	From less than 1 mm to 2 cm (giant molluscum).	From less than 1 mm to 3–5 mm (several centimeters in the confluent lesions).
Lesion surface	Smooth.	Often irregular.
Inflammation	Frequent in individual lesions.	Rare.
Tendency for lesions to become confluent	Extremely rare, though possible on the folds in atopic subjects.	Frequent, producing large plaques, especially in immunocompromised subjects.
Sites involved	Any site; rarely, the inguinal fold in children.	Perianal and perigenital; rarely, the inguinal fold in children.
Clinical course	It regresses spontaneously, approximately within 1 year, with or without inflammation.	The lesions persist for years or decades, but their number changes significantly over time.

Diagnostic Summary

Molluscum contagiosum: hemispheric, translucent papules, sometimes with central depression; they become inflamed easily.
Genital warts: elongated or flat papules, merging in the folds, unlikely to become inflamed.

1. Molluscum Contagiosum

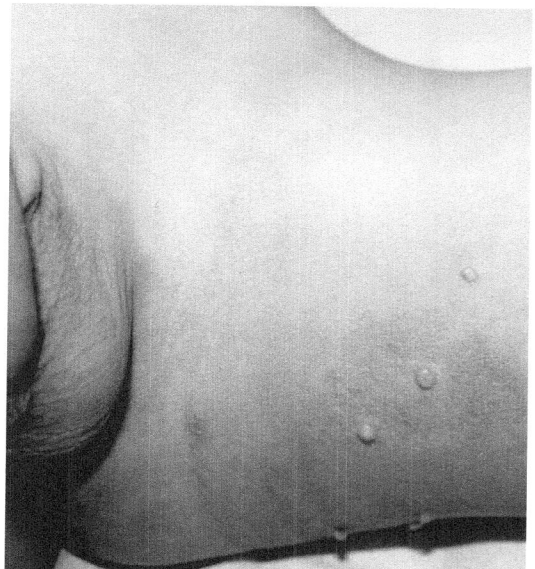

Fig. 1

2. Genital Warts

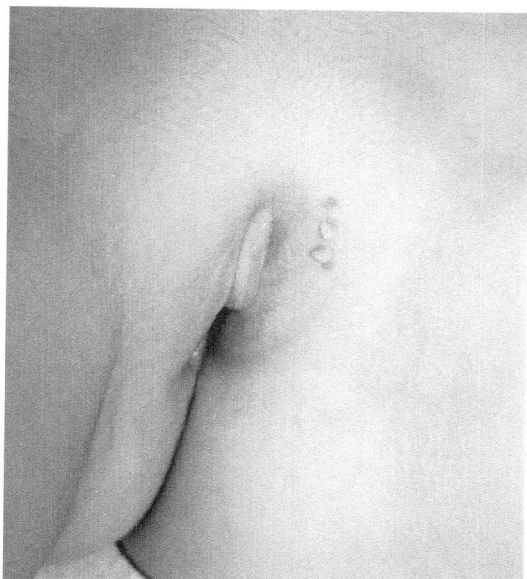

Fig. 2

Bacterial Infections

E. Bonifazi, *Differential Diagnosis in Pediatric Dermatology,*
DOI: 10.1007/978-88-470-2859-3_4 © Springer-Verlag Italia 2013

1. Staphylococcal Scarlet Fever
2. Streptococcal Scarlet Fever

Both *Streptococcus* and *Staphylococcus* [16], thanks to their pyretogenic and vasodilating toxins, can cause fever and generalized skin redness.

	1. Staphylococcal Scarlet Fever	2. Streptococcal Scarlet Fever
Definition	Generalized erythema secondary to staphylococcal infection.	Generalized erythema secondary to streptococcal infection.
Age affected	First five years of life.	From age 4 to 8 years.
Initial focus	Usually cutaneous (pyoderma).	Usually pharyngeal (pharingitis).
Fever	Usually lower than 38.5° C.	Usually higher than 38.5° C.
Enanthem	Usually absent.	Usually present.
Symptoms	Disproportionately more asthenia than fever.	Nausea, headache, and abdominal pain.
Initial cutaneous findings	Cyanotic erythema affecting the eyelids and the perioral region.	Punctate erythema of the chest, perioral pallor.
Rash	Punctate, more marked on the folds.	Punctate, more marked on the folds.
Other clinical findings	Phlyctenas, blisters, pustules, and hypotension.	Perioral pallor, strawberry tongue, petechiae, punctate maculae on the palate, lymphadenopathy of the neck.

> ## Diagnostic Summary
> **Staphylococcal scarlet fever:** initial staphylococcal focus usually affecting the skin, with no involvement of the oral cavity; cyanotic erythema affecting the perioral region.
> **Streptococcal scarlet fever:** streptococcal pharyngitis, strawberry tongue, lymphadenopathy of the neck.

1. Staphylococcal Scarlet Fever

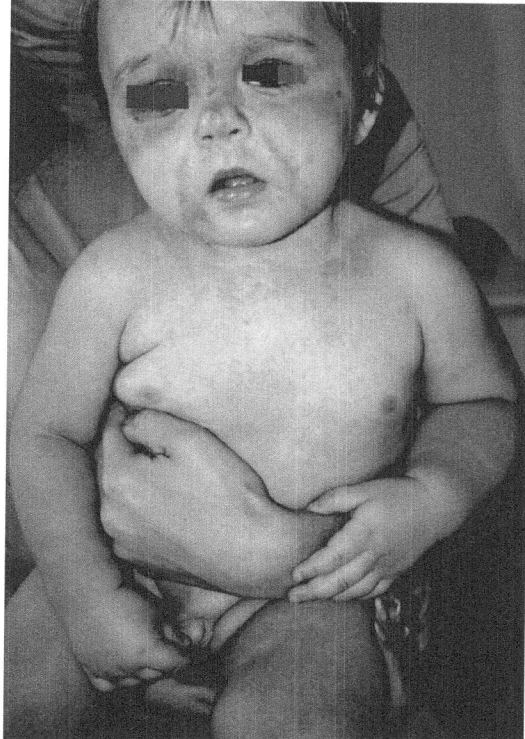

Fig. 1a

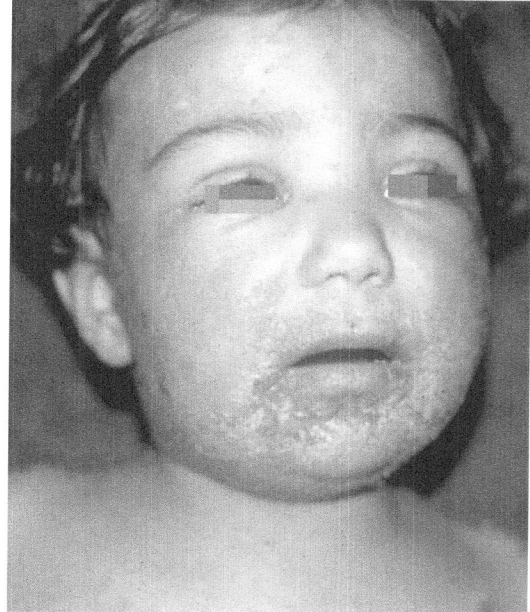

Fig. 1b

2. Streptococcal Scarlet Fever

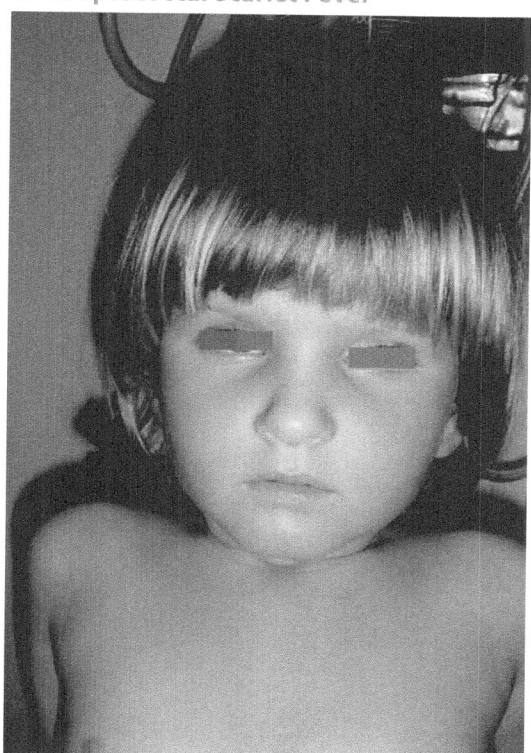

Fig. 2a

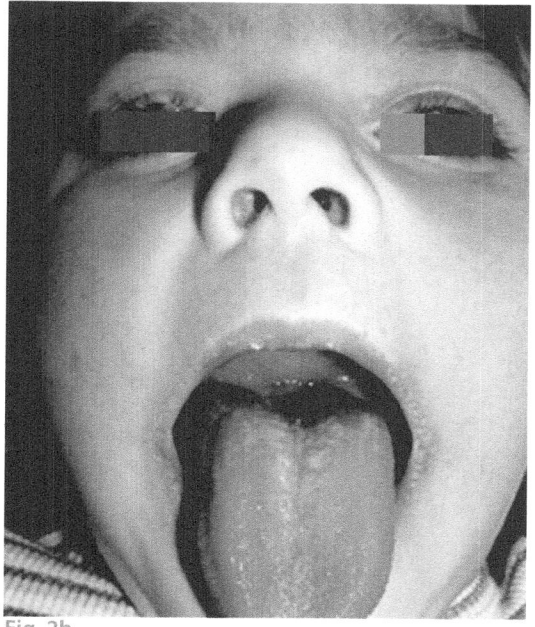

Fig. 2b

Fungal Infections

E. Bonifazi, *Differential Diagnosis in Pediatric Dermatology,*
DOI: 10.1007/978-88-470-2859-3_5 © Springer-Verlag Italia 2013

1. Segmental Vitiligo
2. Hypopigmented Pityriasis Versicolor

White spots unilaterally distributed on the chest can appear for the first time during summertime when reaching peripubertal age. They can be due to segmental vitiligo or hypopigmented pityriasis versicolor.

	1. Segmental Vitiligo	2. Hypopigmented Pityriasis Versicolor
Definition	Disease due to autoimmune destruction of melanin.	Mycotic infection due to the *Malassezia* fungi.
Site of lesions	Limbs, face, chest.	Chest, root of the upper limbs.
Lesion distribution	Unilateral.	Initially asymmetrical, sometimes unilateral.
Lesion size	Variable, ranging from a few centimeters to 30–40 cm.	Ranging from 1 mm to 30–40 cm; smaller lesions are found at the periphery.
Clinical course	It can worsen or improve. However, a complete regression is extremely rare.	It can completely regress or recur yearly.
Effect of the sun	Redness; occasionally, partial repigmentation occurs.	Regression, hypopigmentation.

Diagnostic Summary

Segmental vitiligo: one or few spots with irregular outline, which redden and repigment during the summertime, though they never completely regress.

Hypopigmented pityriasis versicolor: roundish lesions, highly variable in size though smaller at the periphery, which can completely regress or recur periodically.

1. Segmental Vitiligo

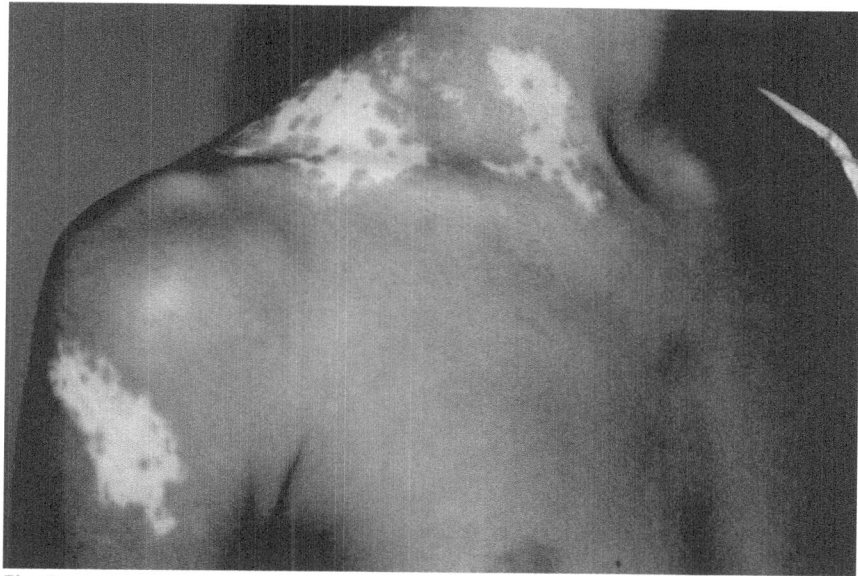

Fig. 1

2. Hypopigmented Pityriasis Versicolor

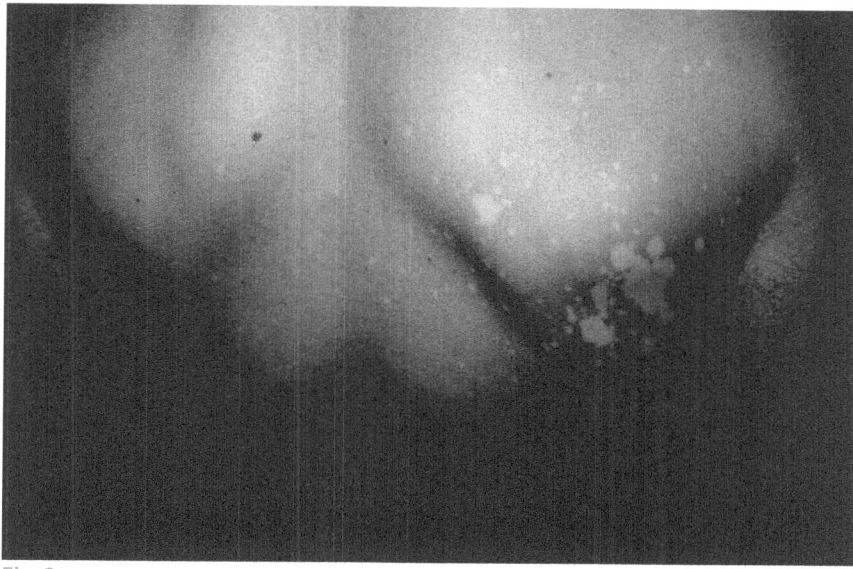

Fig. 2

Parasitic Infestations

E. Bonifazi, *Differential Diagnosis in Pediatric Dermatology*,
DOI: 10.1007/978-88-470-2859-3_6 © Springer-Verlag Italia 2013

1. Nodular Scabies
2. Nodular Mastocytosis

In children, scabies may present, especially at a late stage, only as inflammatory nodules. Mastocytosis may also present as a few nodules, which undergo episodic, urticaria-like inflammation.

	1. Nodular Scabies	2. Nodular Mastocytosis
Definition	Parasitosis caused by a mite.	Benign proliferation of mast cells.
Family history	Other family members started to scratch almost simultaneously.	Usually negative.
Symptoms	Severe itching, usually spasmodic, when the nodules swell.	Mild itching, present only when the nodules undergo urtication.
Flush	Absent.	Often present.
Location of nodules	Characteristic location of scabies: axillary, periumbilical, perigenital.	Usually localized to the chest area.
Duration of nodular inflammation	Hours or days.	10–20 min.
Blister formation on the nodule	Absent.	Frequent.

Diagnostic Summary

Nodular scabies: nodules located where scabies is typically found in children with a family history of recent itching.

Nodular mastocytosis: nodules present since birth with episodes of urtication, blister formation, or erythematous flush.

1. Nodular Scabies

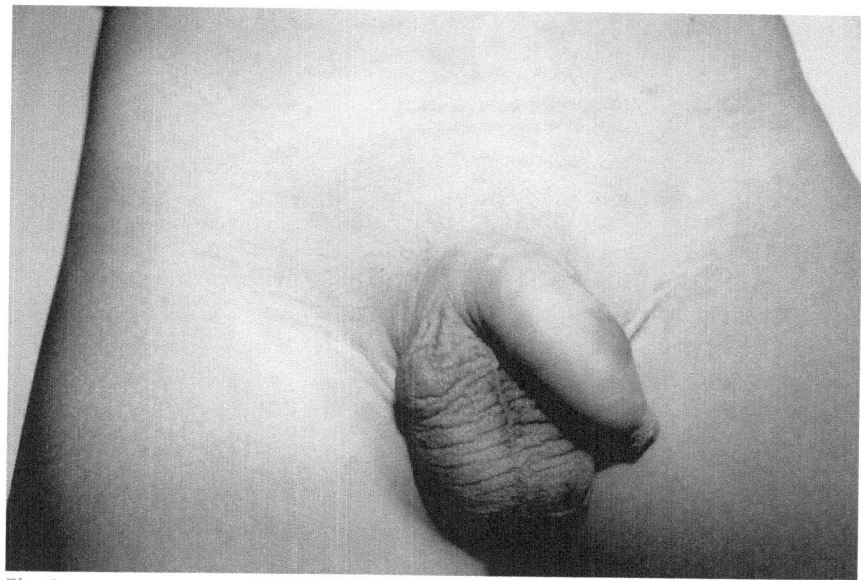

Fig. 1

2. Nodular Mastocytosis

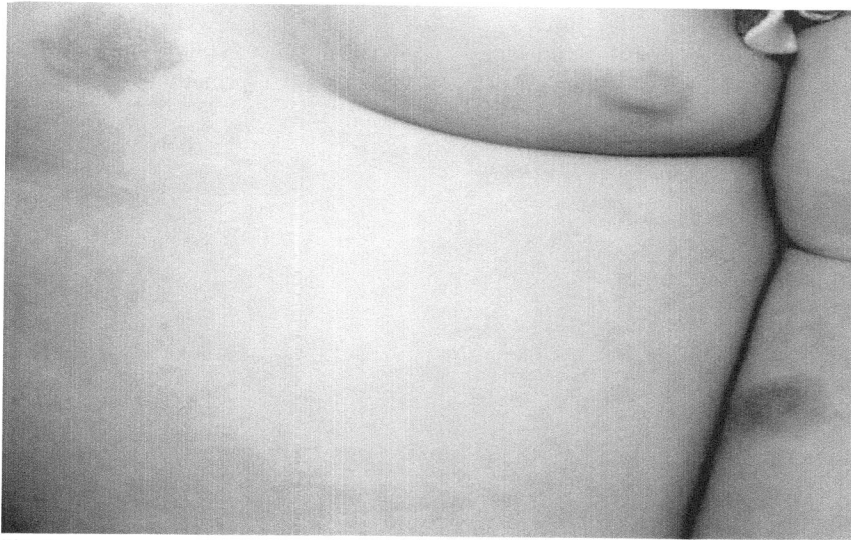

Fig. 2

1. Peripilar Keratin Hair Casts
2. Head Louse Nits

Peripilar keratin hair casts [17] can be reminiscent of head louse nits.

	1. Peripilar Keratin Hair Casts	**2. Head Louse Nits**
Definition	Cylindrical structures made of keratin, which are the remnants of the epithelial sheaths enveloping the hairs in the pilar duct inside the skin.	Eggs of *Pediculus humanus capitis*.
Prevalence	Rare.	Frequent.
Shape	Cylindrical (Fig. 1b).	Pyriform (Fig. 2b).
Length	Variable, from 1 to 4 mm.	Uniform, about 1 mm.
Dermoscopy	The cylinder envelops the hair like a sleeve (Fig. 1b).	The nit is firmly stuck to the hair, like a flag to its flagpole (Fig. 2b).
Sliding along the hair shaft	Easily accomplished; the hair casts easily slide along the hair shaft.	The nits resist sliding along the hair shaft, especially when viable.

Diagnostic Summary

Peripilar keratin hair casts: they have varying length and slide along the hair shaft.
Head louse nits: they have uniform length and stick firmly to the hair shaft.

1. Peripilar Keratin Hair Casts

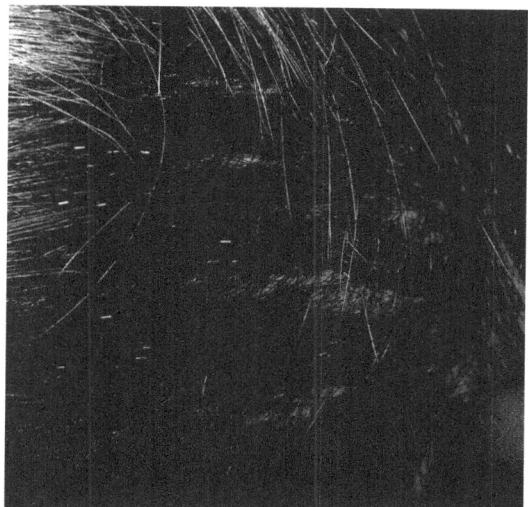

Fig. 1a

2. Head Louse Nits

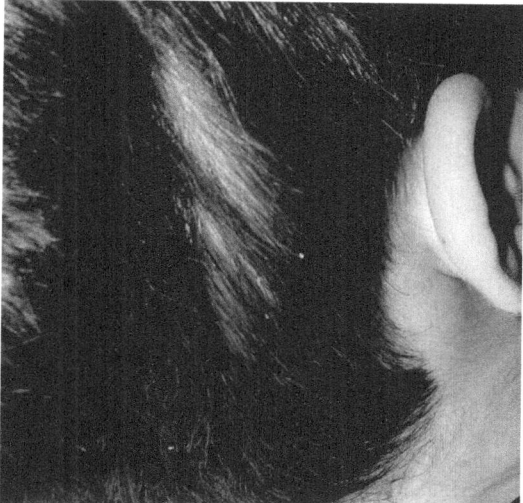

Fig. 2a

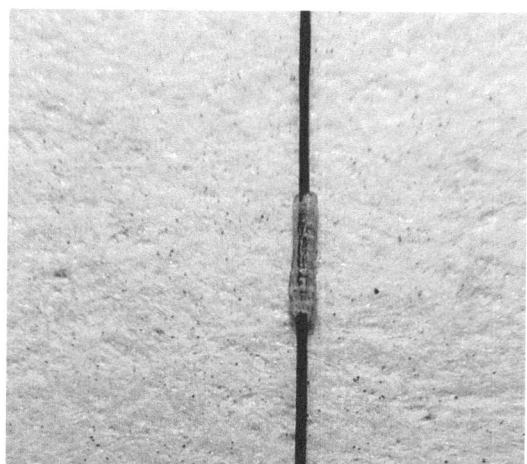

Fig. 1b Hair cast, 30x, dermoscopy

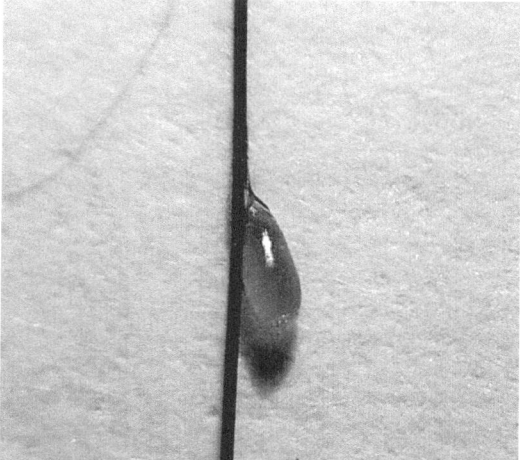

Fig. 2b Viable nit, 30x, dermoscopy

1. Pediculosis Palpebrarum
2. Atopic Blepharitis

Pediculosis palpebrarum can simulate atopic blepharitis, thus making differential diagnosis difficult.

	1. Pediculosis Palpebrarum	**2. Atopic Blepharitis**
Definition	Infestation with crab lice (*Phthirus pubis*), which in children affects the eyelashes. The parasite lays the eggs at the follicular opening, i.e., where the eyelashes exit from the skin.	Inflammation of the free border of the eyelids. In children, it is an expression of atopic diathesis, which is sometimes associated with atopic conjunctivitis.
Frequency	Rare.	More frequent.
Age affected	Prepubertal period.	First decades of life.
Symptoms	Asymptomatic, at least initially.	Intense itching, foreign body sensation.
Moving lice	Sometimes visible (Fig. 1).	Absent.
Nits	Always present.	Absent.
Dry scales	Usually absent.	Always present.
Erythema of the free border	Usually absent.	Sometimes present.
Other sites affected	Hairline behind the auricle; blue spots (maculae ceruleae) on the chest.	Sometimes the conjunctiva, especially the tarsal/palpebral conjunctiva.
Clinical course	Acute, until it is diagnosed.	Chronic-recurrent for months or years.

Diagnostic Summary

Pediculosis palpebrarum: recent onset, nits on the eyelashes, blue spots (maculae ceruleae).
Atopic blepharitis: longer history, itching, lack of nits.

1. Pediculosis Palpebrarum

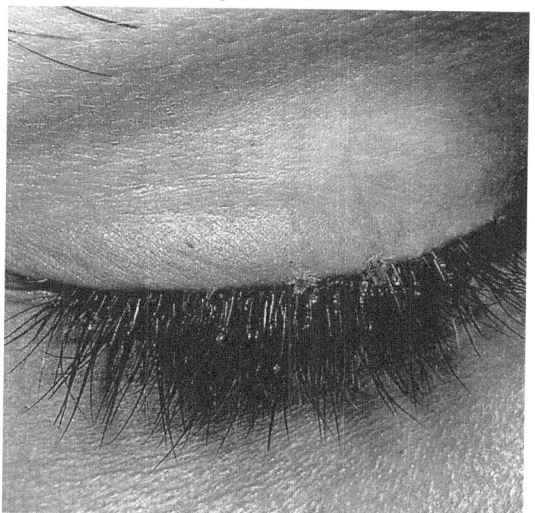

Fig. 1

2. Atopic Blepharitis

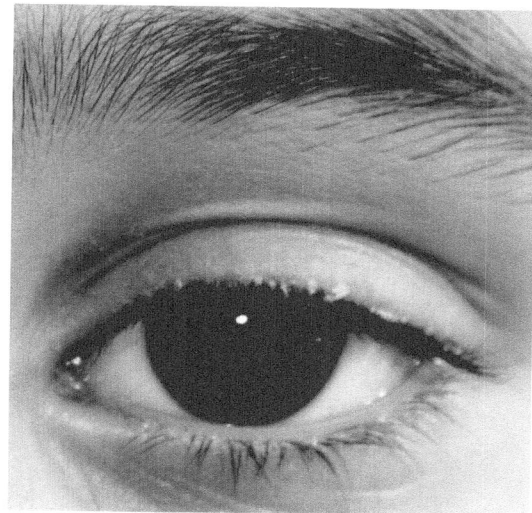

Fig. 2

Acne

E. Bonifazi, *Differential Diagnosis in Pediatric Dermatology,*
DOI: 10.1007/978-88-470-2859-3_7 © Springer-Verlag Italia 2013

1. Acne
2. Angiofibromas of Tuberous Sclerosis

Angiofibromas of tuberous sclerosis, which are characteristically localized around the nose, can look like the papular lesions of acne and should therefore be differentiated from this condition.

	1. Acne	**2. Angiofibromas of Tuberous Sclerosis**
Definition	A disease of the pilosebaceous unit, due to genetic factors and hormonal changes, characterized by comedones and inflammatory lesions of various type.	Angiofibromas are benign tumors characteristic of tuberous sclerosis, an inherited skin disorder characterized by skin and neurological lesions.
Time of onset	Puberty.	First decade of life.
Location of skin lesions	Cheeks, forehead, back.	Perinasal region.
Lesion size	From 1 mm to 2 cm.	From 1 to 5–6 mm.
Lesion type	Comedones, inflammatory papules, pustules, nodules.	Reddish papules.
Inflammation	Usually present.	Absent.
Clinical course of individual lesions	Individual inflammatory lesions subside in days or weeks.	Stable over time.
Duration	A few years.	Progressive worsening throughout life.
Other cutaneous findings	Absent.	Congenital white spots, Koenen tumors, fibrous plaque, shagreen patches.
Neurological involvement	Absent.	Usually seizures.
Response to treatment	It improves with anti-acne medical therapy.	They improve with topical rapamycin treatment [18].

Diagnostic Summary

Acne: acquired disease usually occurring at puberty, characterized by polymorphic lesions.
Angiofibromas of tuberous sclerosis: congenital disease that begins before puberty and lasts throughout life; it is characterized by monomorphic angiofibromas localized to the face.

1. Acne

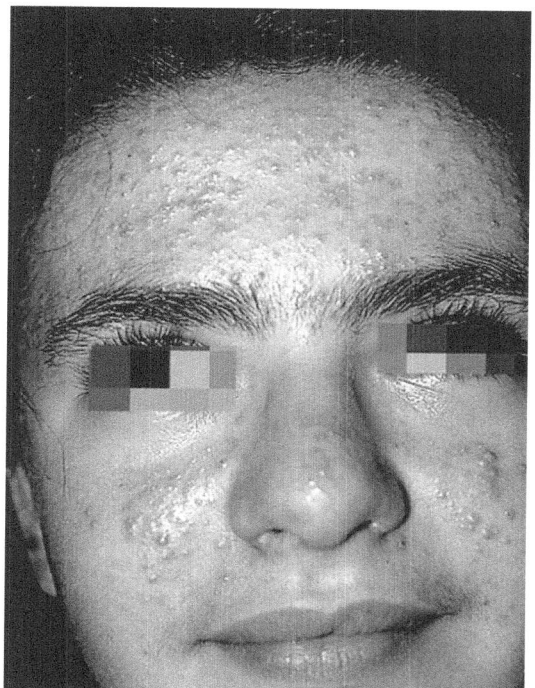

Fig. 1

2. Angiofibromas of Tuberous Sclerosis

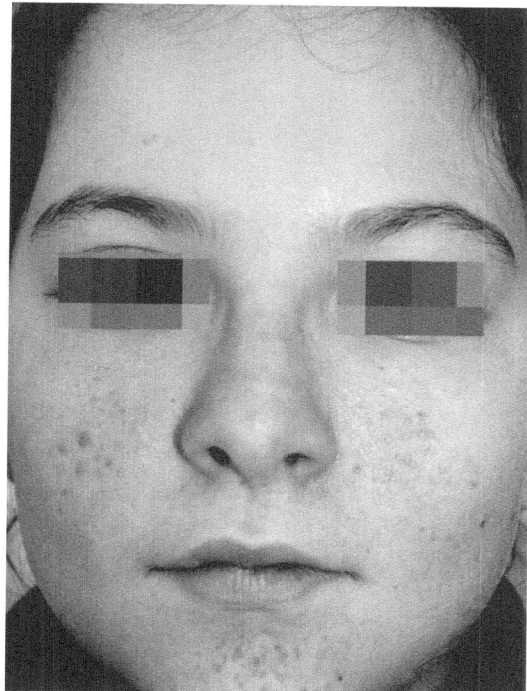

Fig. 2

Allergic Diseases

E. Bonifazi, *Differential Diagnosis in Pediatric Dermatology,*
DOI: 10.1007/978-88-470-2859-3_8 © Springer-Verlag Italia 2013

1. Atopic Dermatitis
2. Dermatitis Herpetiformis

Intensely itchy, chronic inflammatory lesions in children are usually due to atopic dermatitis. Rarely, they can be caused by dermatitis herpetiformis, the first and most classical extraintestinal manifestation of celiac disease.

	1. Atopic Dermatitis	**2. Dermatitis Herpetiformis**
Definition	It is the dermatitis of subjects with a family and/or personal history of atopy.	It is the dermatitis that usually occurs in people with celiac disease.
Prevalence	12.8% of all pediatric diseases [5].	0.1% of all pediatric diseases [5].
Time of onset	At any age, the first 6 months of life in more than 50% of cases.	The infantile form begins after the second year of life.
Case history	Personal and/or family history of atopic disease in more than 70% of cases.	Positive personal and/or family history of autoimmune diseases.
Itching	Severe, with periodic changes.	Severe, persistent.
Lesion type	Eczematous.	Characteristic erythematous and infiltrated lesions, with flat surface, circinate, with vesicles usually barely visible.
Lesion distribution	The face in the first year of life, the flexor surface of the elbows and knees later on.	Centripetal, with prevalent involvement of the chest— especially the scapular region and the root of the limbs, especially a triangular area of the extensor surface of the forearm with its basis on the elbow.
Laboratory tests	Skin prick test for atopy often positive.	Autoantibodies against endomysium and transglutaminases.
Response to a gluten-free diet	Never.	Almost always in children.

Diagnostic Summary

Atopic dermatitis: eczematous lesions localized to the folds of the elbows and knees.
Dermatitis herpetiformis: erythematous-infiltrated circinate lesions of the shoulder girdle and extensor region of the elbow.

1. Atopic Dermatitis

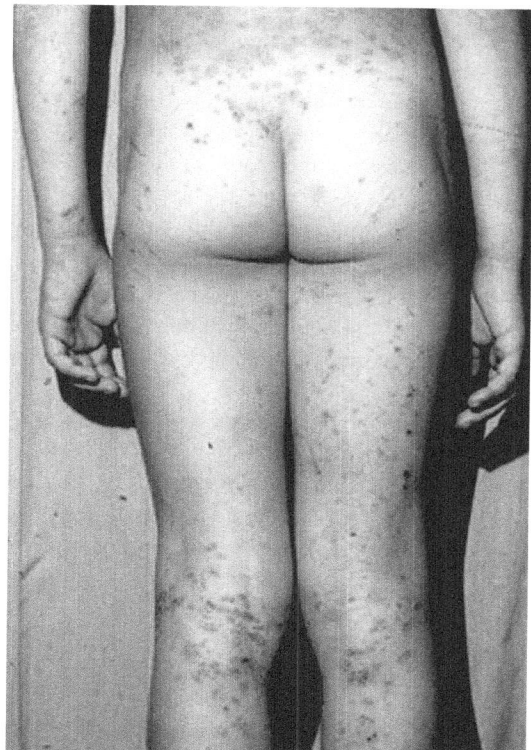

Fig. 1

2. Dermatitis Herpetiformis

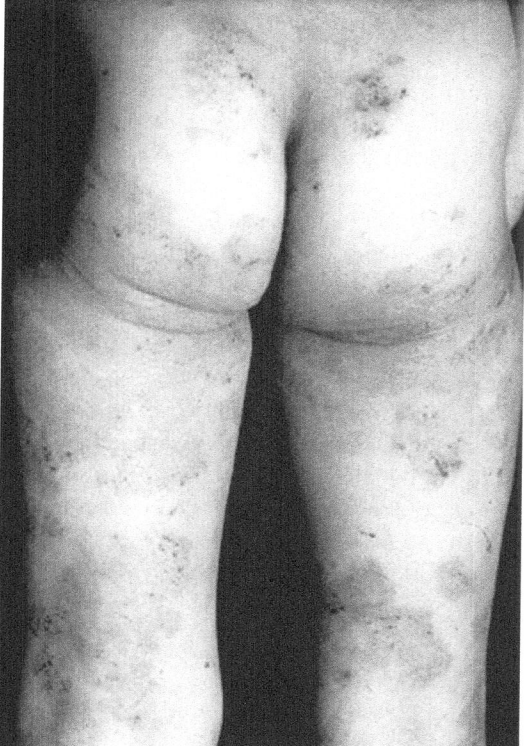

Fig. 2

1. Hypopigmented Atopic Dermatitis
2. Hypopigmented Pityriasis Versicolor

Any inflammatory disease that affects the epidermis and superficial dermis from late spring through to early fall can be responsible for hypopigmented sequelae. Atopic dermatitis is not exempt from this rule and being the most frequent dermatitis in children, it is by far the most common cause of hypopigmented sequelae in children.

On the other hand, in adults, although present, atopic dermatitis has a lower incidence and therefore the most common cause of hypopigmented sequelae is pityriasis versicolor (so called because it has hyper- and hypopigmented lesions), a superficial fungal infection due to the *Malassezia* yeasts. These fungi have a characteristic lipophilia, which is why pityriasis versicolor is less frequent in children, whose low androgen levels mean that they cannot stimulate sebaceous secretions; consequently, pityriasis versicolor is rare in children.

The very frequent association between pityriasis versicolor and hypopigmented sequelae in adults, has given rise to the assumption that all hypopigmented lesions have a fungal origin. This assumption is responsible for an excessive and unjustified consumption of antimycotic drugs. The increasing prescribing of oral antimycotic drugs could also be responsible for systemic side effects. Such an assumption should not include children, since pityriasis versicolor is rare in children.

	1. Hypopigmented Atopic Dermatitis	2. Hypopigmented Pityriasis Versicolor
Definition	Dermatitis of atopic subjects.	Mycotic infection due to the *Malassezia* yeasts.
Prevalence	High in children, low in adults.	Low in children, high in adults.
Lesion location	Cheeks, limbs, more rarely the chest.	Chest and root of upper limbs in adults. Forehead and parotid region in children.
Lesion distribution	Usually symmetrical.	Initially asymmetrical, sometimes monolateral.
Lesion size	2–3 cm, uniform.	From 1 mm to 30–40 cm; smaller lesions are found in the periphery.
Lesion outline	Blurred.	Clearly defined.
Mycological examination	Negative.	Positive.

Diagnostic Summary

Hypopigmented atopic dermatitis: frequent in children, it is prevalent on the face and limbs; it is usually symmetrical with blurred borders.

Hypopigmented pityriasis versicolor: rare in children, where it mainly affects the forehead; it is asymmetrical with clearly defined borders.

1. Hypopigmented Atopic Dermatitis

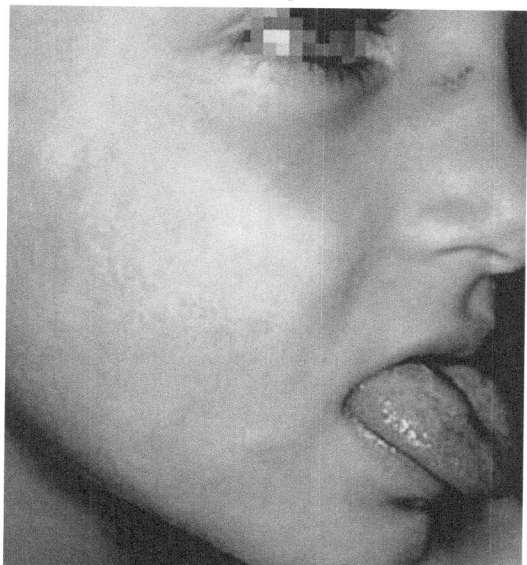

Fig. 1

2. Hypopigmented Pityriasis Versicolor

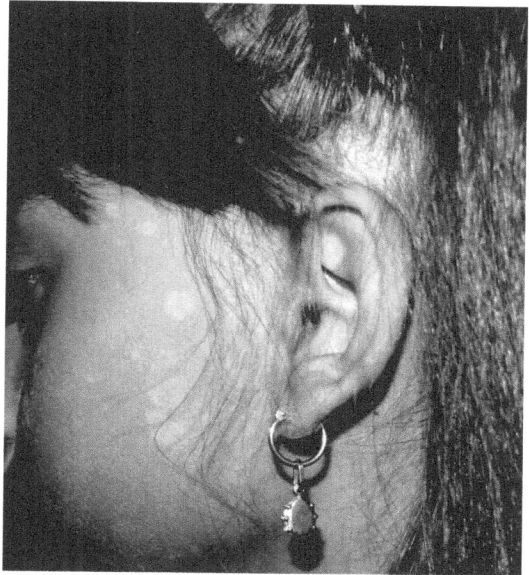

Fig. 2

1. Hypopigmented Atopic Dermatitis
2. Systemic Vitiligo

Systemic vitiligo, which symmetrically affects the skin, must be differentiated from the hypopigmented sequelae of atopic dermatitis.

	1. Hypopigmented Atopic Dermatitis	2. Systemic Vitiligo
Definition	It is the most frequent dermatitis of atopic subjects.	Autoimmune disease which causes the destruction of melanin.
Family history	Positive for atopic diseases.	Positive for autoimmune diseases.
Lesion color	Lighter than normal skin.	White.
Scaling	Often present.	Absent.
Lesion outline	Blurred.	Clearly defined.
Follicular repigmentation	Absent.	Sometimes present.
Sun-induced redness of lesions	Absent.	Present.
Clinical course of lesions in winter	Regression.	Persistence with minor evidence.

Diagnostic Summary

Hypopigmented atopic dermatitis: often scaling lesions with blurred borders.
Systemic vitiligo: lesions with well-defined borders; on sun exposure, they redden and sometimes undergo repigmentation.

1. Hypopigmented Atopic Dermatitis

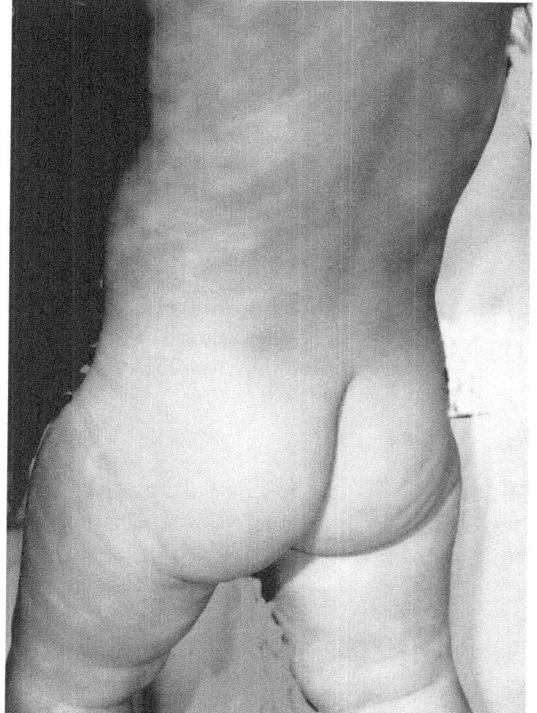

Fig. 1

2. Systemic Vitiligo

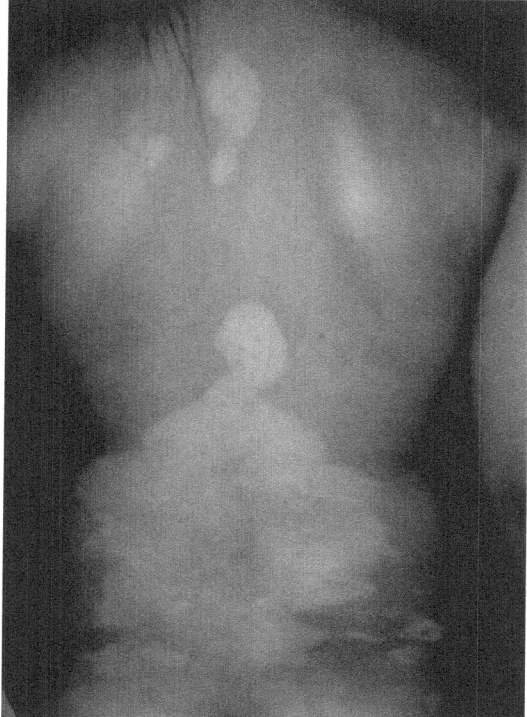

Fig. 2

1. Atopic Dermatitis
2. Tinea Faciei

The differential diagnosis between atopic dermatitis and tinea faciei generally does not arise because the two diseases have different clinical features. However, in some cases, the differential diagnosis between these two diseases may be problematic.

	1. Atopic Dermatitis	2. Tinea Faciei
Definition	It is the dermatitis characteristic of an atopic constitution.	Superficial infection of the epidermis caused by dermatophytes [13].
Itching	Usually present.	Usually absent.
Facial location	Face in the first year of life, later on the eyelid and perioral regions, except in severe cases when it can affect the entire face.	As it is an exposed area, the face is one of the most frequent initial sites of tinea.
Lesion type	Scaling, erythematous and scaling, exuding.	Erythematous and scaling, rarely with micropustules.
Lesion asymmetry	Rare.	Frequent.
Lesion outline	Generally blurred.	Clearly defined.
Tendency to central resolution	Absent.	Present.

Diagnostic Summary

Atopic dermatitis: itchy lesions, with blurred borders, usually symmetrical.
Tinea faciei: asymmetrical lesions, with clearly defined borders and central resolution.

1. Atopic Dermatitis

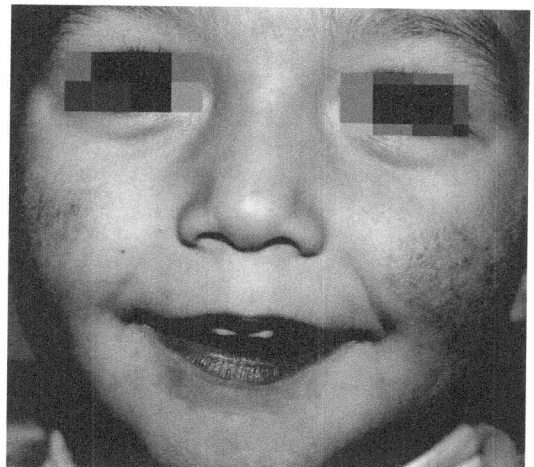

Fig. 1a

2. Tinea Faciei

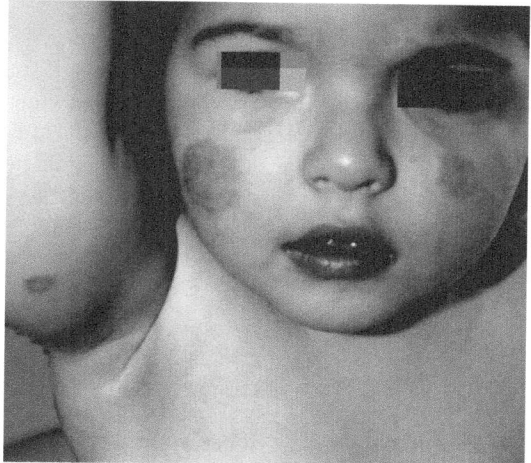

Fig. 2a

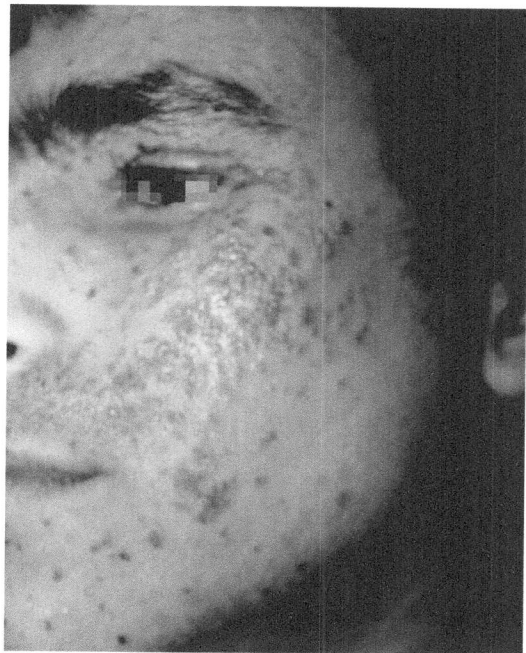

Fig. 1b

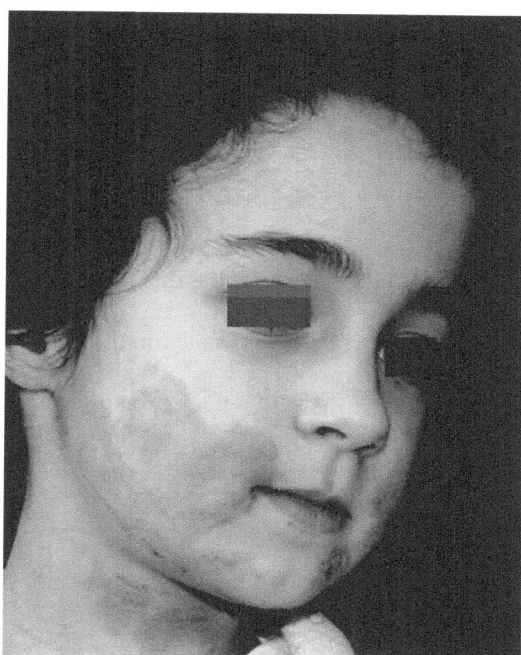

Fig. 2b

1. Atopic Dermatitis
2. Scalp Psoriasis

Atopic dermatitis and psoriasis are the most frequent causes of scaling dermatitis of the scalp in the pre-pubertal period. When the scalp is the only site affected, the diagnosis is made more difficult by the presence of hair, which makes the physical examination less simple, and by the physiological characteristics of the scalp, which is the common denominator of the two different skin disorders, in this case making erythema less visible and scaling more evident.

	1. Atopic Dermatitis	2. Scalp Psoriasis
Time of onset	Usually, the first months of life.	Any age.
Family history	Positive for dermatitis or other atopic manifestations.	Positive for psoriasis or other autoimmune disorders.
Itching	Present, usually severe.	Absent or light.
Facial involvement	Frequent on the cheeks in the first year, later affecting the periocular and perioral areas.	Rare, except for the frontal limit of the hairline.
Lesion outline	Poorly outlined.	Clearly defined.
Exudation	It can be present, especially in the first months of life.	Absent.
Scaling	Usually thin.	Multilayered.
Scratching lesions	Often present.	Absent.

Diagnostic Summary

Atopic dermatitis: it begins early in life, is associated with itching, and its lesions have poorly defined borders.
Scalp psoriasis: lesions are scarcely symptomatic, with clearly defined borders, and are characterized by massive hyperkeratosis.

1. Atopic Dermatitis

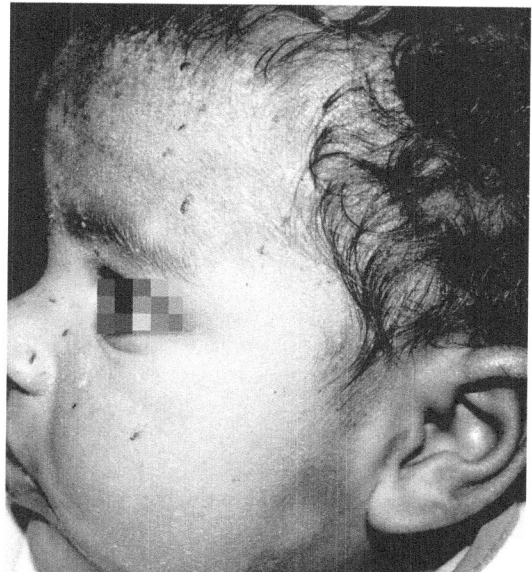

Fig. 1

2. Scalp Psoriasis

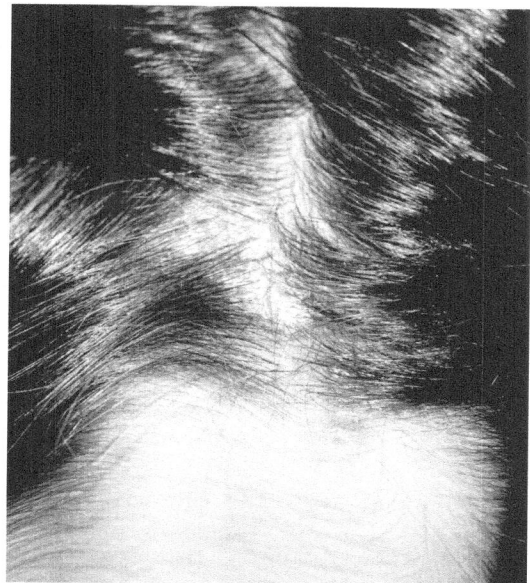

Fig. 2

1. Keratosis Pilaris Rubra
2. Atopic Dermatitis

Keratosis pilaris is a disorder genetically transmitted by an autosomal dominant trait, characterized by hyperkeratosis of the follicular openings, i.e., the external orifices of the pilosebaceous follicles. When keratosis is associated with marked perifollicular erythema, we talk about about keratosis pilaris rubra [19]. This condition must be differentiated from atopic dermatitis.

	1. Keratosis Pilaris Rubra	2. Atopic Dermatitis
Definition	Inherited skin disorder characterized by follicular keratosis and perifollicular erythema.	Dermatitis characteristic of the atopic subject.
Time of onset	Usually, within the first year of life.	Usually, within the first year of life.
Summer improvement	Present.	Present.
Lesion duration on the cheeks	Decades.	First years of life, even later on in the most severe cases.
Itching	Usually absent.	Usually present.
Lesion location	Cheeks with eyelids, forehead, and chin spared.	Cheeks, eyelids, forehead, and chin in the first year, later on the eyelids and perioral region.
Other sites affected	Follicular keratosis of the lateral surface of the arms.	Folds, especially cubital and popliteal.
Lesion morphology	Punctate hyperkeratosis surrounded by erythema, without exudation, crusts, and scales.	Confluent erythema, scales, crusts, sometimes exudation.
Facial coloration	Persistent rubeosis of the cheeks.	After the first year of life, the pallor of the cheeks contrasts with the erythematous lesions of the eyelids and perioral region.

Diagnostic Summary

Keratosis pilaris rubra: punctate lesions, non-itchy, sparing the eyelids.
Atopic dermatitis: confluent erythematous and crusted lesions that are itchy and affect the eyelids.

1. Keratosis Pilaris Rubra

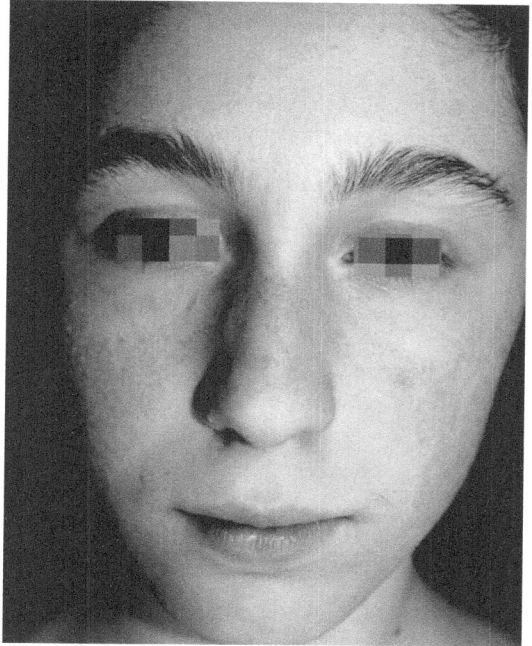

Fig. 1a

2. Atopic Dermatitis

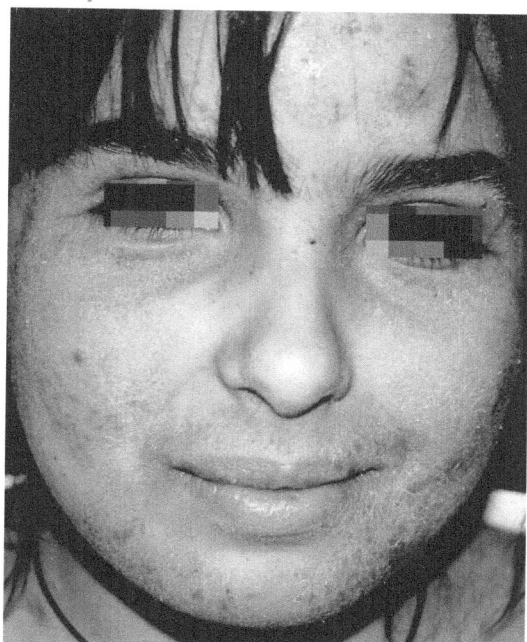

Fig. 2a

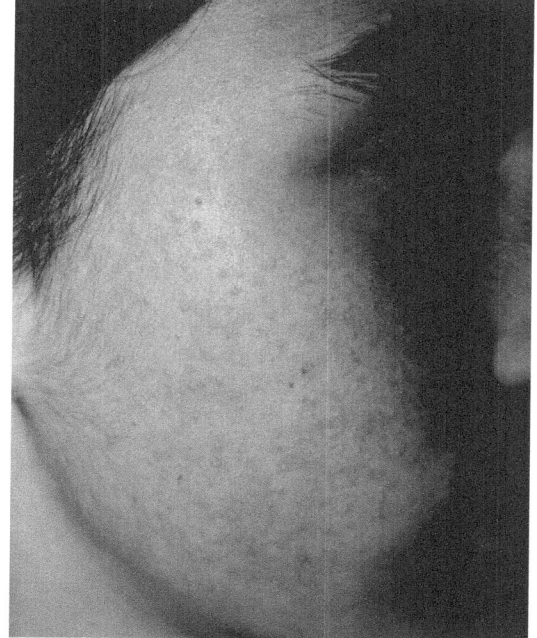

Fig. 1b

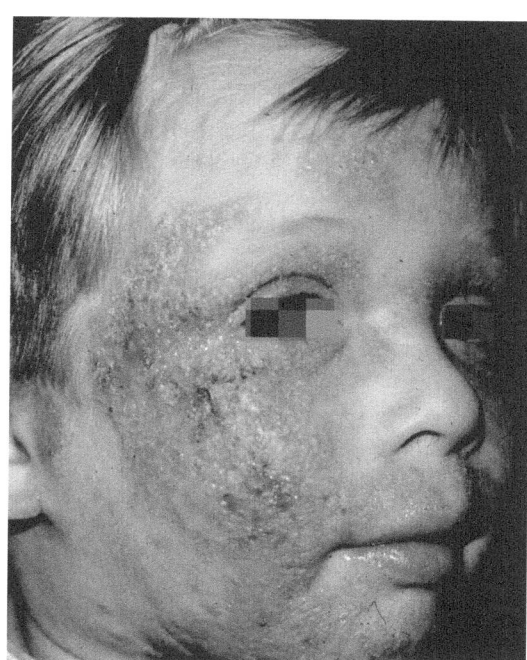

Fig. 2b

1. Early Atopic Dermatitis
2. Neonatal Acne

In the second month of life, the two most common diseases that affect the child's face are atopic dermatitis and neonatal acne, which are very different from each other in terms of pathogenesis and clinical course.

	1. Early Atopic Dermatitis	**2. Neonatal Acne**
Definition	Dermatitis characteristic of the atopic subject.	Skin disease due to androgenic stimulation of the pilosebaceous follicle.
Difference between the sexes	No difference.	Prevalent in males.
Itching	Present in the more severe cases and highlighted by rubbing against a pillow, restlessness, and sleeplessness.	Absent.
Lesion location	Cheeks, forehead.	Cheeks, rarely the forehead.
Lesion distribution	Confluent lesions; isolated lesions may be observed only in the initial phase.	Isolated lesions.
Lesion type	Scaling, erythematous and scaling, exuding.	Comedones, papules, pustules.
Lesion duration	Many months.	Usually, a few weeks.
Sequelae	None.	Atrophic scars when the lesions are larger than 3 mm.

Diagnostic Summary

Early atopic dermatitis: symptomatic eczematous lesions, usually confluent.
Neonatal acne: asymptomatic, isolated comedones, papules, and pustules.

1. Early Atopic Dermatitis

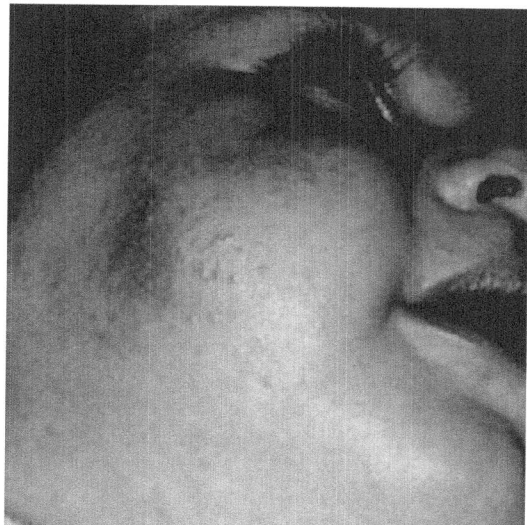

Fig. 1

2. Neonatal Acne

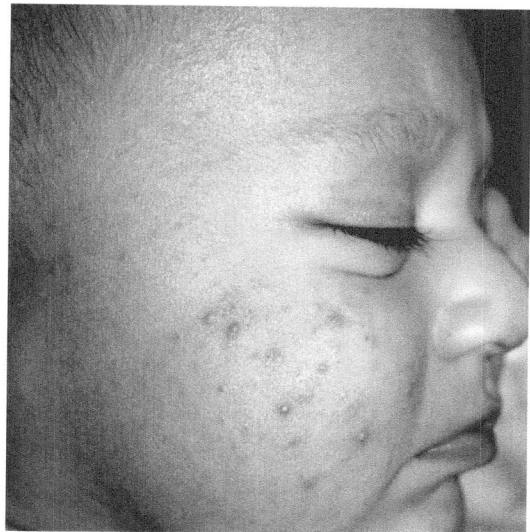

Fig. 2

1. Atopic Dermatitis
2. Scabies

Atopic dermatitis and scabies are very different diseases in all respects, but share a symptom, i.e., itching, which can be the symptom of disease onset and/or the reason why the child comes to be examined. The diagnosis of atopic dermatitis is usually easy, but some difficulty may be encountered in the early stages of life given the lack of the typical chronic-recurrent course and when sites other than the classical ones are affected. The diagnosis of scabies is rather difficult, sometimes even for the skilled physician.

	1. Atopic Dermatitis	**2. Scabies**
Definition	It is the most frequent dermatitis in atopic subjects.	Skin infestation from *Sarcoptes scabiei* var. *hominis*.
Prevalence	It is the most frequent cause of itching in children, mainly in the first years of life.	Highly variable depending on the socioeconomic conditions and the historical period (war, immigration).
Familial itching	Only one person in the family is affected. When two family members are affected, one of them has usually been affected for a much longer period.	Several relatives may be affected and may have started to scratch themselves more or less at the same time.
Gross nodules	May be observed in adults (prurigo nodularis), but are rarely found in children.	Often present in children at the primary locations for scabies.
First sites to be affected	In the first year, the scalp and cheeks, sparing the diaper area. From the second year onwards, the flexor surface of the elbows and knees (Fig. 1b).	Interdigital spaces and the ulnar region of the hand; wrist (flexor aspect), elbow (extensor aspect), armpit, navel, buttocks, groin area, penis, primary and secondary genitalia in adults, foot and rarely head in the first year of life (Fig. 2b).
Specific lesions	Eczematous, exuding or erythematous and scaling.	1-mm-wide, 1-cm-long furrows at the primary location for scabies.
"Ex adiuvantibus" criterion	Significant improvement after the application of topical corticosteroids. Acaricides applied erroneously can worsen dermatitis and itching.	Significant improvement of itching after the first acaricide treatment. Corticosteroids applied erroneously do not relieve itching.

1. Atopic Dermatitis

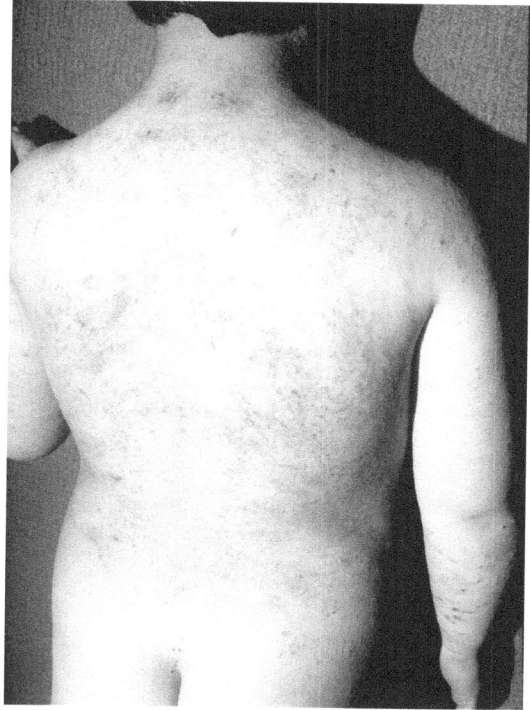

Fig. 1a

2. Scabies

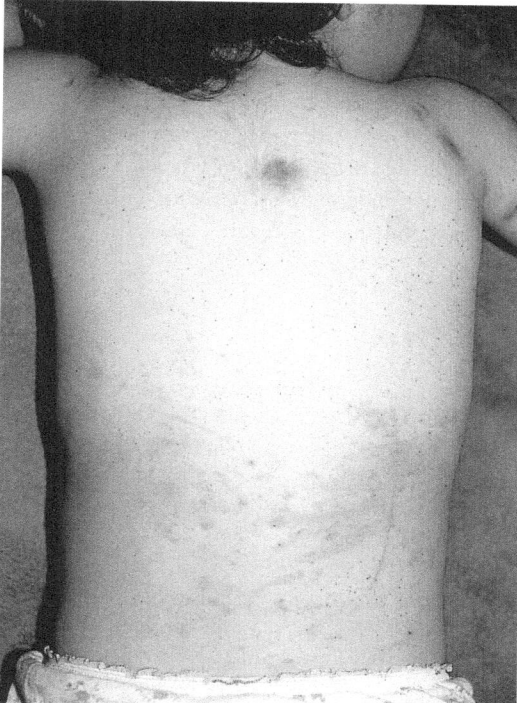

Fig. 2a

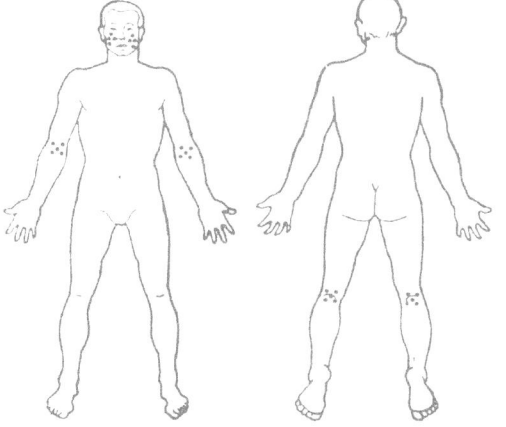

Fig. 1b Atopic dermatitis: affected sites

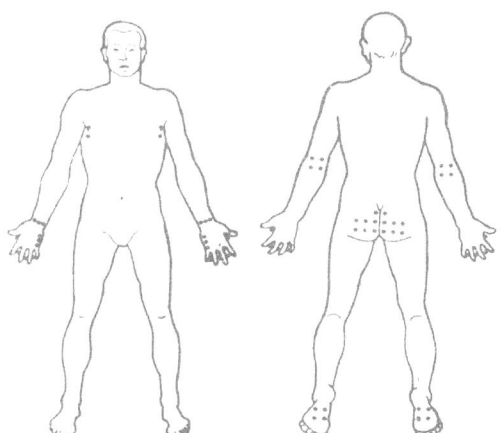

Fig. 2b Scabies: affected sites

Diagnostic Summary

Atopic dermatitis: it starts and is prevalent on the head in the first year of life; later on, it affects the flexor surface of the elbows and knees; it improves significantly with topical corticosteroids.
Scabies: concurrent itching in several family members, involvement of the primary locations for scabies, recovery with acaricides.

1. Fixed Drug Eruption
2. Recurrent Herpes Simplex

Fixed drug eruption and recurrent herpes simplex (HS) are very different diseases. However, they share one characteristic: they always recur at the same site. The former recurs when the child is again given the responsible drug, the latter when the virus is reactivated. Unfortunately, both eventualities occur almost always under the same conditions, i.e., when the child has an infection of the upper respiratory tract that is accompanied by fever.

	1. Fixed Drug Eruption	2. Recurrent Herpes Simplex
Definition	Disease caused by an allergic reaction to a drug.	Secondary, recurrent infection due to HSV.
Lesion location	Periorificial regions, hands.	Any site, in children usually a cheek.
Number of lesions	Multiple, often far from one another.	Multiple, close to one another.
Lesion type	Erythema, serum-filled blisters.	Erythema, vesicopustules, crusts.
Lesion size	From 1 cm to several decimeters.	1–2 mm.
Sequelae	Dusky violaceous, persistent.	Slight, transient discoloration.
Recurrence	It recurs until the cause is identified and removed.	It recurs for many years and is not influenced by drugs.
Sites of recurrence	The previous ones, to which other, new sites can be added.	The previous ones or sites nearby the previous ones.
Laboratory tests	Oral challenge.	Tzanck smear to identify balloon cells, polymerase chain reaction.

Diagnostic Summary

Fixed drug eruption: when retaking the offending drug, the violaceous sequelae redden; lesions from 1 cm to several decimeters, even distant from one another.
Recurrent herpes simplex: vesicopustules in clusters, usually to 1–3 mm in size.

1. Fixed Drug Eruption

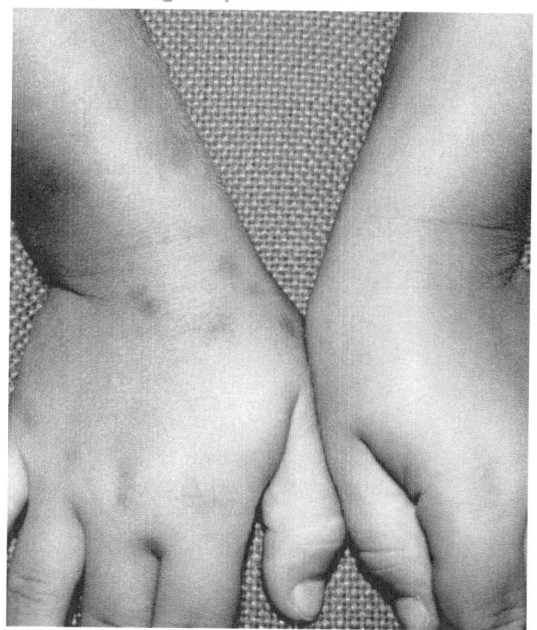

Fig. 1a

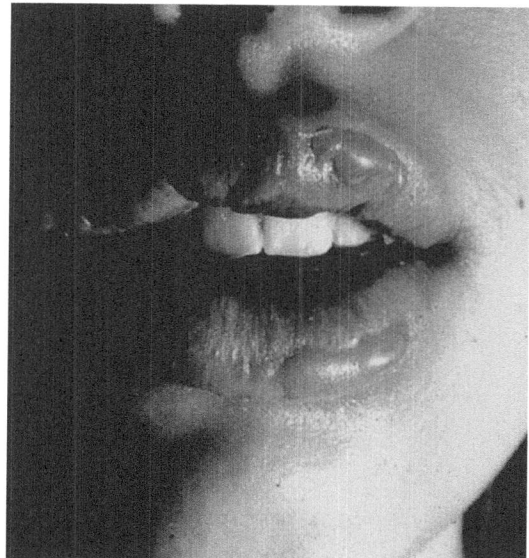

Fig. 1b

2. Recurrent Herpes Simplex

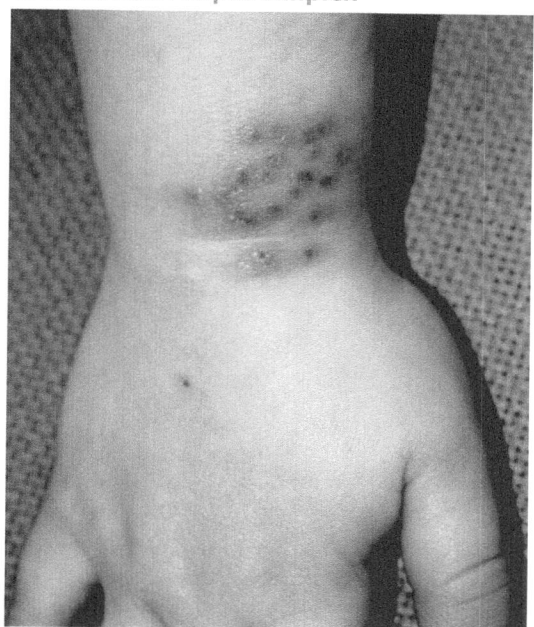

Fig. 2a

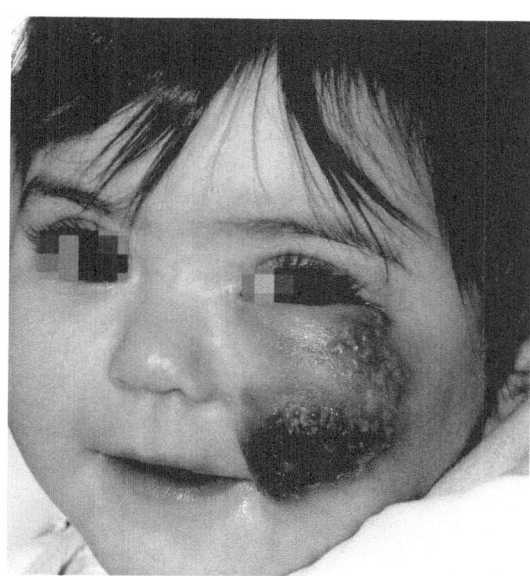

Fig. 2b

1. Drug-Induced or Viral Epidermal Necrolysis
2. Staphylococcal Scalded Skin Syndrome

Epidermal necrolysis is characterized by the coming away of large patches of the epidermis due to the action of exfoliating "toxins" that, by spreading through the blood, widely affect the skin. Its causes, as usual in dermatology, can be multiple, though they are mainly viral, pharmacological, and staphylococcal. The viral and staphylococcal forms are most frequent and severe in children: the differential diagnosis between the two forms is vital to establish a correct antibiotic therapy in the staphylococcal form [20].

	1. Drug-Induced or Viral Epidermal Necrolysis	2. Staphylococcal Scalded Skin Syndrome
Definition	Epidermal necrolysis caused by drugs or viruses.	Epidermal necrolysis due to *Staphylococcus aureus*.
Initial findings	Inflammation of the upper respiratory tract, flu-like syndrome.	Pyoderma, conjunctivitis, vulvovaginitis, other suppurative foci.
Eye involvement	Hemorrhagic inflammation, possible residual synechiae.	A suppurative conjunctivitis can be an initial focus.
Oral involvement	Frequent.	Absent.
Lesion morphology	Blisters arise on an initially punctate rash. Sequelae of the latter can always be seen at the periphery of the confluent lesions.	Blisters arise on uniformly erythematous or apparently healthy skin.
Histology	Dermo-epidermal cleavage.	Intraepidermal cleavage.
Response to antibiotics	None.	Excellent, when early.

Diagnostic Summary

Drug-induced or viral epidermal necrolysis: frequent ocular and oral involvement, the blisters arise on a punctate skin rash.
Staphylococcal scalded skin syndrome: staphylococcal initial focus, the blisters arise on normal or uniformly erythematous skin.

1. Drug-Induced or Viral Epidermal Necrolysis

2. Staphylococcal Scalded Skin Syndrome

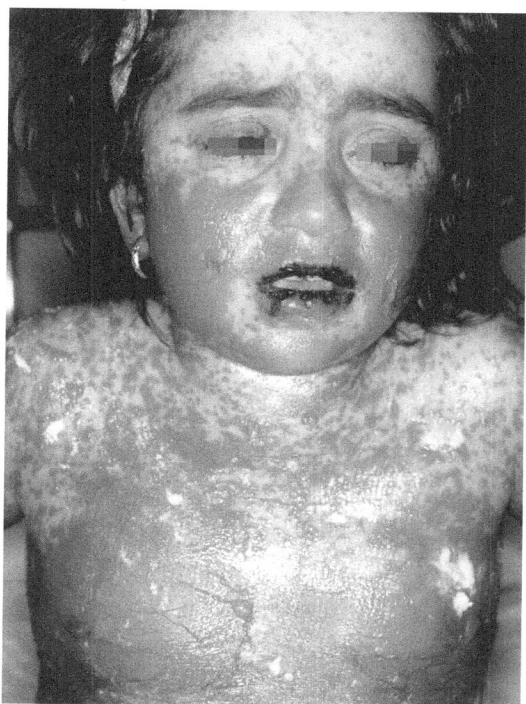

Fig. 1a

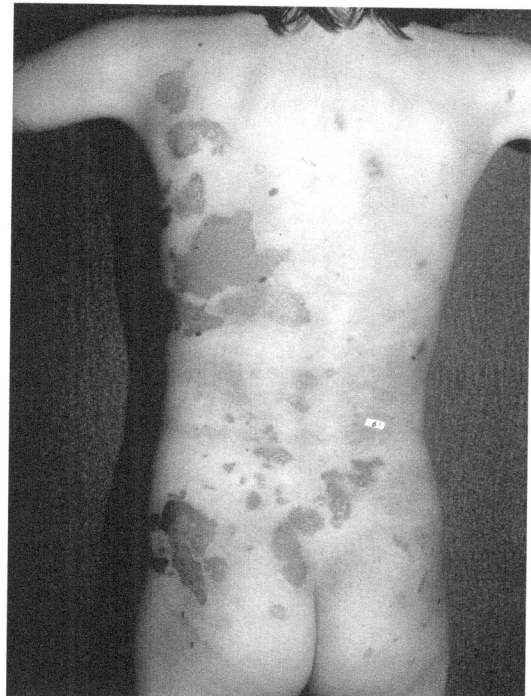

Fig. 2a

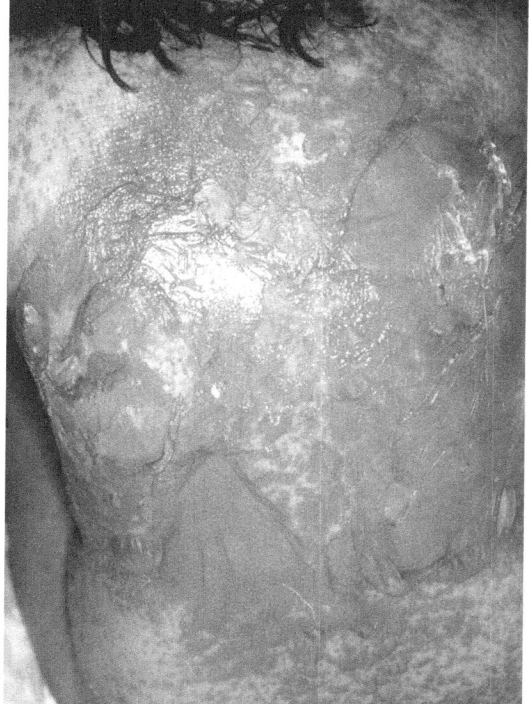

Fig. 1b

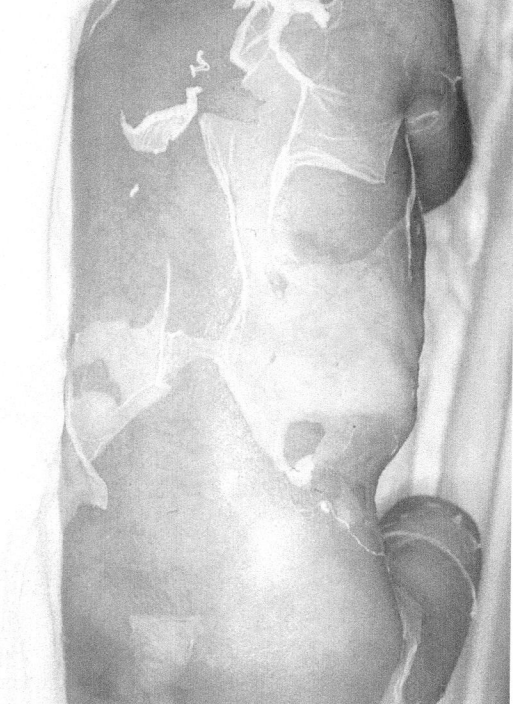

Fig. 2b

1. Henoch–Schönlein Purpura
2. Gianotti–Crosti Syndrome

Henoch–Schönlein purpura and papular acrodermatitis of childhood (Gianotti–Crosti syndrome) are both characterized by a purpuric acrolocated papular eruption and therefore must be differentiated from each other.

	1. Henoch–Schönlein Purpura	2. Gianotti–Crosti Syndrome
Definition	Small-vessel vasculitis with immunoglobulin A-mediated involvement of the skin, kidney, joints, and gastrointestinal tract.	Papular eruption secondary, in most cases, to infection with hepatotropic viruses.
Time of onset	Usually the first decade of life, from the third year onwards.	Mainly in the first decade.
Lesion distribution	Lower limbs, forearms.	Face, limbs, buttocks, rarely the chest.
Clinical features	Polymorphic erythematous papules often associated with urticarial or necrotic lesions.	Monomorphic gross papules of uniform diameter, close to one another but nonconfluent.
Purpuric lesions	Always present.	Occasionally present, especially on the legs due to compression stimuli.
Clinical course	Usually, recurrent episodes for 4–8 months.	Single eruption that disappears in 3–5 weeks with mild scaling.
Laboratory tests	Hematuria.	Increased levels of transaminases.
Other findings	Arthralgias, vomiting, abdominal pain.	Hepatosplenomegaly, generalized adenopathy.

Diagnostic Summary

Henoch–Schönlein purpura: orthostatic polymorphic eruption with hematuria, and abdominal and joint pain.

Gianotti–Crosti syndrome: monomorphic acrolocated papular eruption often associated with hypertransaminasemia.

1. Henoch–Schönlein Purpura

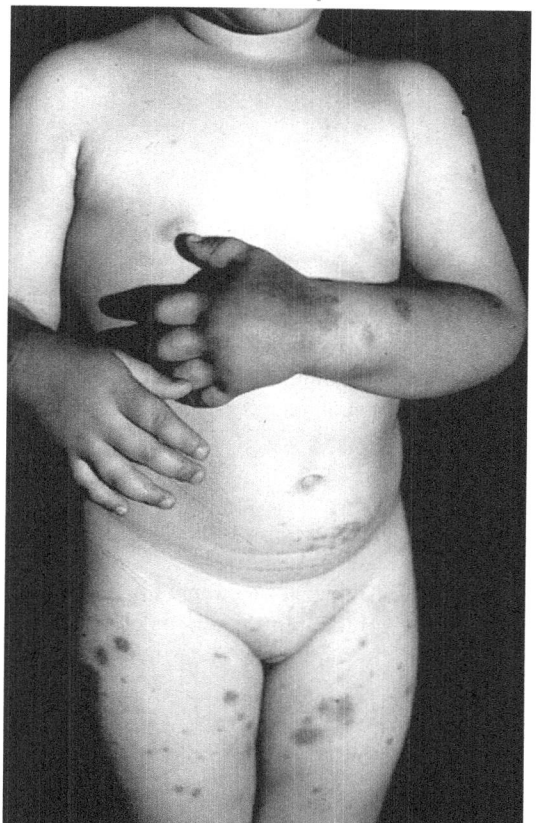

Fig. 1

2. Gianotti–Crosti Syndrome

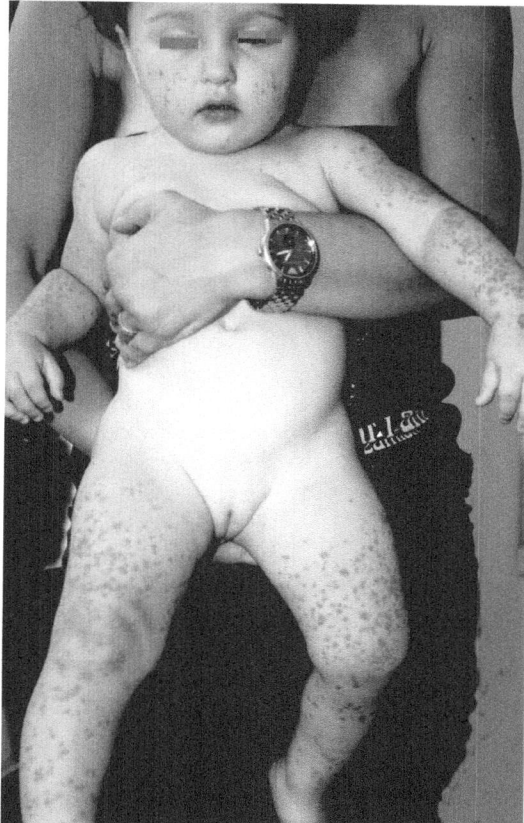

Fig. 2

1. Henoch–Schönlein Purpura
2. Hemorrhagic Urticaria

Both Henoch–Schönlein purpura and hemorrhagic urticaria may present wheals and bruises, thus making a differential diagnosis necessary.

	1. Henoch–Schönlein Purpura	2. Hemorrhagic Urticaria
Definition	Immunoglobulin A immune complex vasculitis of small vessels affecting the skin and other organs, especially the joints, kidney, and intestine.	Disease linked to the increased permeability of skin capillaries with multiple etiology, allergic or nonallergic.
Time of onset	After 2 years, with a peak between 4 and 7 years.	Any age, even from the first few months of life.
Other organs to be affected	Joints, kidney, intestine; more rarely others, such as the eye, nervous system, and so on.	Transient functional impairment of the joints when the wheals are located in the periarticular region.
Lesion morphology	Edema, wheals, hemorrhagic papules, ecchymotic nodules, crusted lesions.	Wheals, followed by superficial bruises, which reproduce the shape and size of the wheals.
Duration of individual lesions	Dependent on the type of lesion; nevertheless, a matter of days.	Hours for the wheals, 2–3 days for the bruises.
Total duration of eruption	4–8 months.	From days to months.
Lesion distribution	Lower limbs, with greater involvement of the legs than the thighs, buttocks, and hands.	Everywhere on the body.

Diagnostic Summary

Henoch–Schönlein purpura: subacute vasculitis with polymorphic lesions in orthostatic sites.
Hemorrhagic urticaria: wheals and bruises, the latter reproducing the form of the wheals at any site.

1. Henoch–Schönlein Purpura

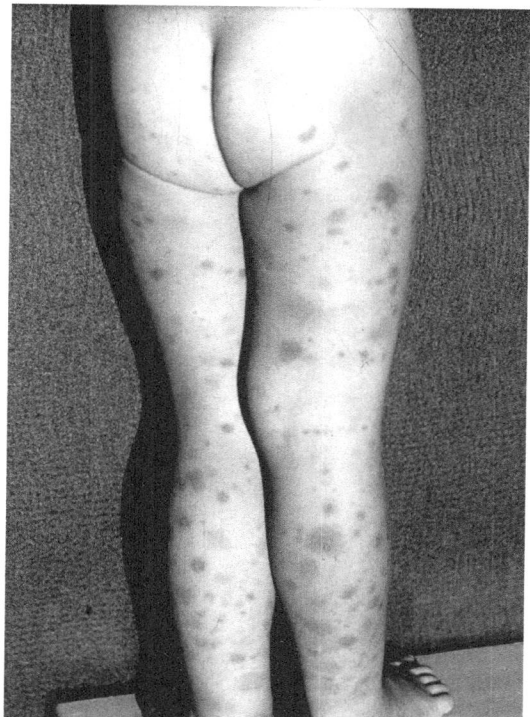

Fig. 1

2. Hemorrhagic Urticaria

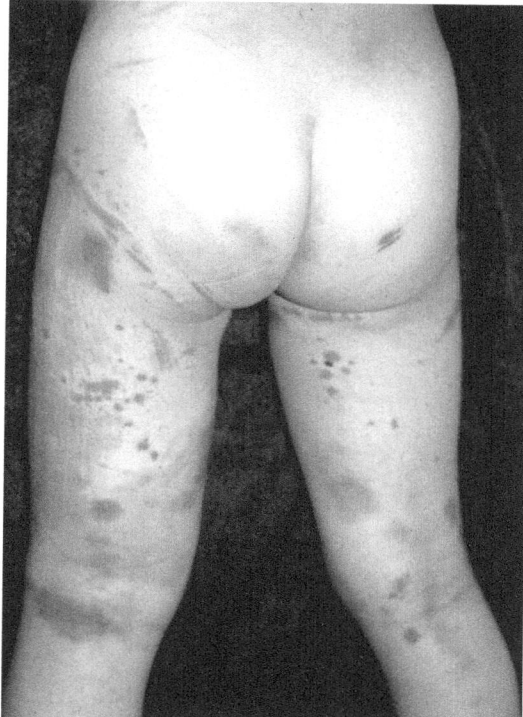

Fig. 2

Autoimmune Skin Disorders

E. Bonifazi, *Differential Diagnosis in Pediatric Dermatology,*
DOI: 10.1007/978-88-470-2859-3_9 © Springer-Verlag Italia 2013

1. Diaper Psoriasis
2. Extensive Atopic Dermatitis

In the first two years of life both psoriasis and atopic dermatitis may present with exensive skin lesions, thus giving rise to problems of differential diagnosis.

	1. Diaper Psoriasis	2. Extensive Atopic Dermatitis
Prevalence	0.2% of pediatric skin diseases [5].	12% of pediatric skin diseases [5].
Itching	Absent.	Intense.
Modalities of spreading	Psoriasis appears explosively, weeks or months after the start of a diaper rash.	When atopic dermatitis tends to become generalized, it is accompanied by slow progression of the lesions.
Primary affected site	Diaper area.	Usually, the face in the first year.
Focus of greatest intensity	Diaper area.	Face, folds of the elbows and knees, usually sparing the diaper area.
Lesion type	The secondary lesions have clearly defined borders as in guttate psoriasis. With time, they extend centrifugally and can affect most of the skin surface.	Erythematous lesions with blurred borders, sometimes weeping, which may affect most of the skin surface. More often, weeping is localized to the face and limbs.
Clinical course	The secondary lesions enlarge and then fade to regress in 4–12 weeks; usually, they do not recur.	The lesions are characterized by alternating periods of improvement and worsening and can last months or years.

Diagnostic Summary

Diaper psoriasis: it is not itchy and starts from the diaper area where the lesions are more congested.
Extensive atopic dermatitis: it is itchy and affects first and most severely the face, either sparing or only marginally involving the diaper area.

1. Diaper Psoriasis

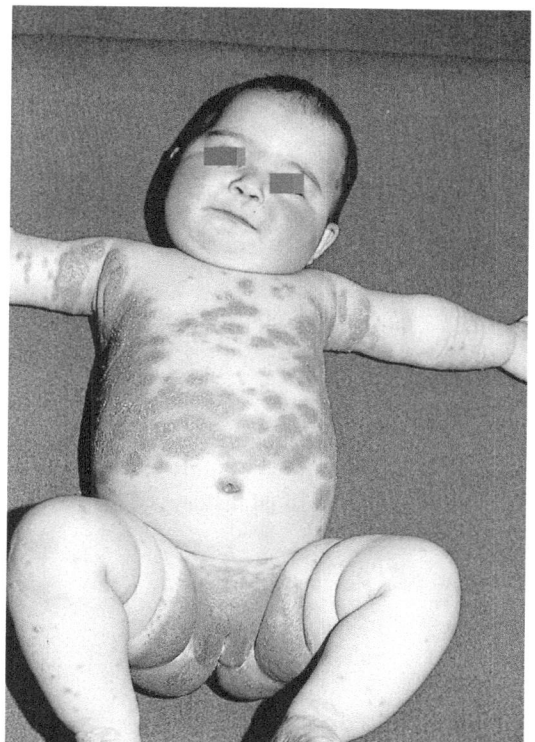

Fig. 1

2. Extensive Atopic Dermatitis

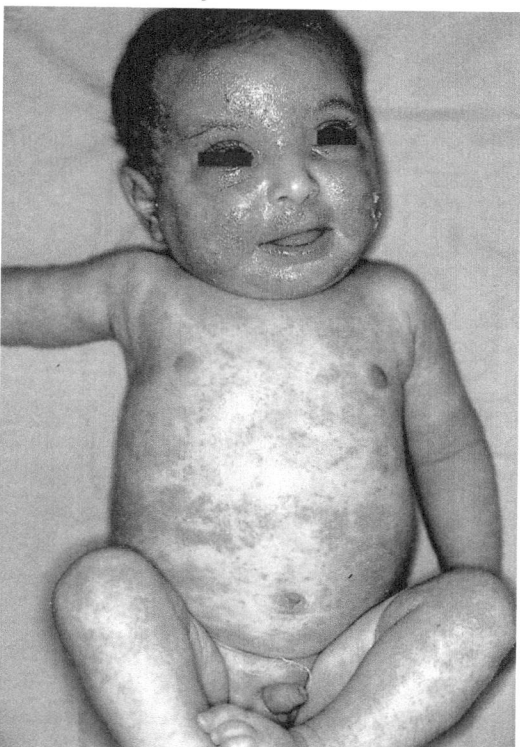

Fig. 2

1. Perigenital Psoriasis
2. Perigenital Atopic Dermatitis

In continent children, both inverse psoriasis and atopic dermatitis may be located, sometimes exclusively, in the perigenital region, thus making differential diagnosis difficult.

	1. Perigenital Psoriasis	2. Perigenital Atopic Dermatitis
Perigenital location	In inverse psoriasis, representing 14% of all cases of psoriasis in children [21].	Rare in atopic dermatitis.
Case history	Familial psoriasis in 25% of cases. Sometimes, a history of atopy coexists.	Atopy (asthma, rhinitis, dermatitis) in family and personal history.
Itching	Mild or absent.	Intense.
Location	Inguinal folds.	Penis, scrotum, vulva, and inguinal folds.
Clinical features	Non-weeping, erythematous lesions, with clearly defined borders.	Erythematous lesions, with blurred borders, which sometimes weep.
Other affected sites	Axillary folds and medial palpebral commissures, occasionally the extensor surface of the limbs.	Cubital and popliteal folds.
Nail involvement	In 30% of cases, pitting or other nail disorders.	Only in the case of eczematous lesions of the matrix.
Clinical course	Chronic.	Chronic-recurrent.

Diagnostic Summary

Perigenital psoriasis: non-itchy lesions with clearly defined borders.
Perigenital atopic dermatitis: itchy lesions with blurred borders.

1. Perigenital Psoriasis

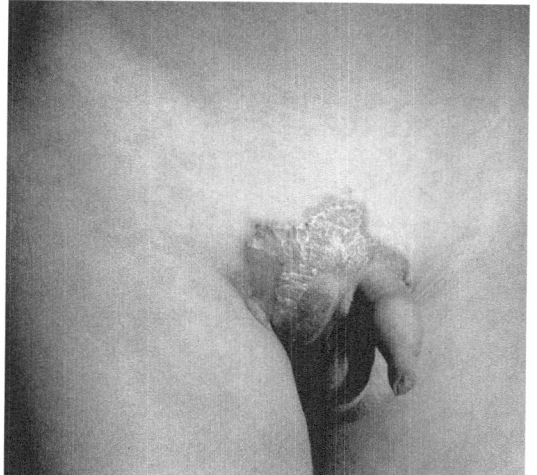

Fig. 1a

2. Perigenital Atopic Dermatitis

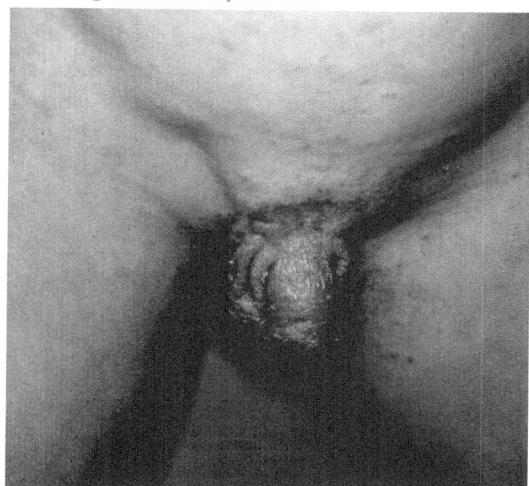

Fig. 2a

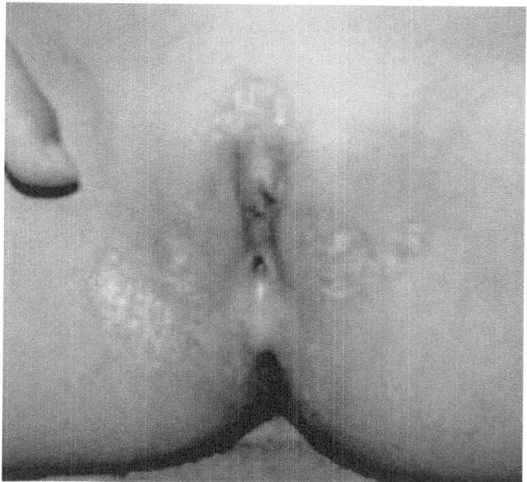

Fig. 1b

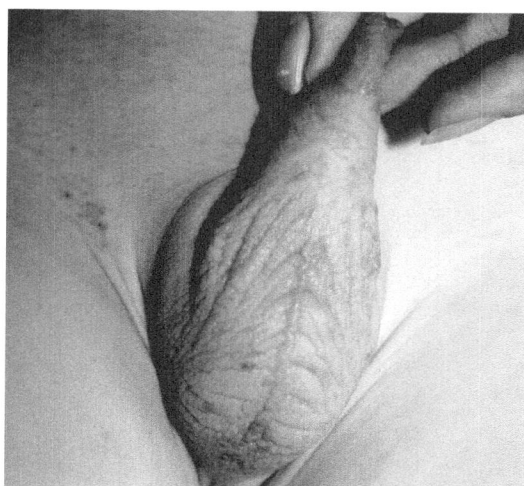

Fig. 2b

1. Pityriasis Rubra Pilaris
2. Follicular Psoriasis

Pityriasis rubra pilaris is rarer in children compared to the more common follicular psoriasis; the latter can simulate the former, thus making a differential diagnosis necessary.

	1. Pityriasis Rubra Pilaris	2. Follicular Psoriasis
Time of onset	Rarely congenital, it usually appears after the first 5 years.	Exceptionally congenital, it may begin at any age.
Palmoplantar keratoderma	Except for the localized form, in which it may be missing, it is practically constant.	Rare.
Scalp involvement	Furfuraceous, nonadherent scaling.	Adherent scales.
Islands of normal skin	Even when erythroderma is present, there are islands of normal skin.	Rare.
Nails	Thickened, but not dystrophic, without yellowish spots.	Often dystrophic with yellow-brown spots.

Diagnostic Summary

Pityriasis rubra pilaris: palmar-plantar keratoderma; no adherent scales on the scalp and fingernails are thickened but without yellowish spots.
Follicular psoriasis: scales adhere to the scalp, nails have yellowish spots, and palmar-plantar keratoderma is absent.

1. Pityriasis Rubra Pilaris

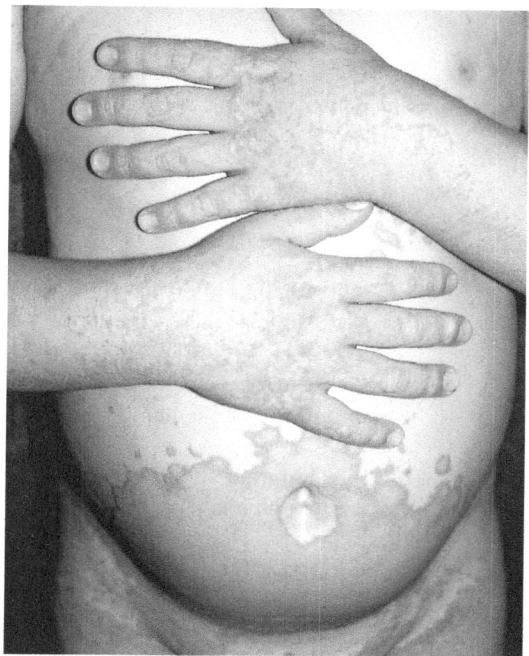

Fig. 1a

2. Follicular Psoriasis

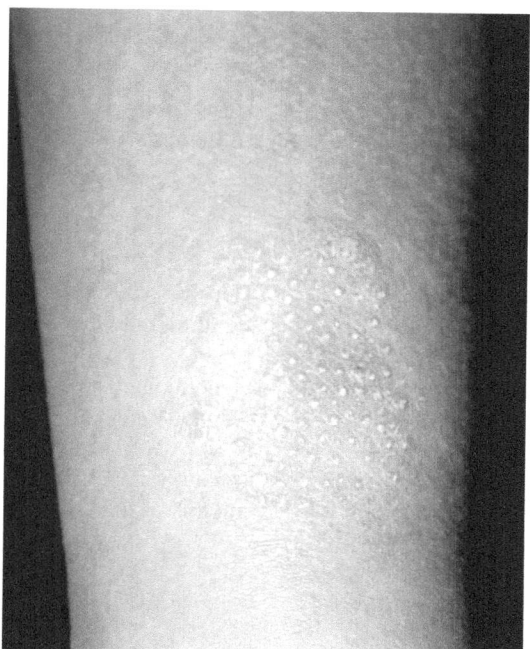

Fig. 2a

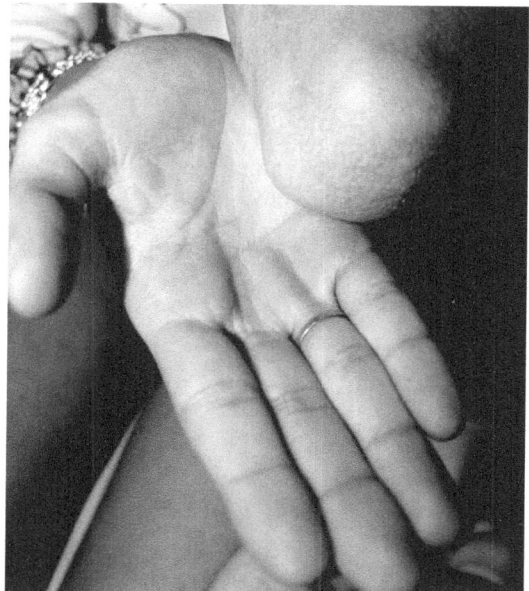

Fig. 1b

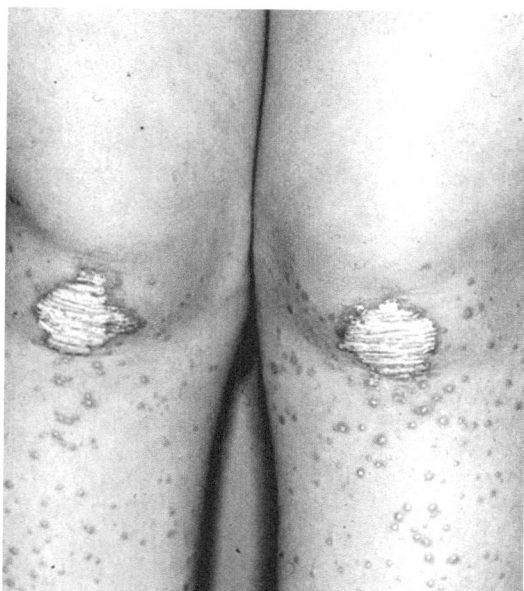

Fig. 2b

1. Alopecia Areata
2. Trichotillomania

A patch of alopecia with perfectly normal scalp skin can occur both in alopecia areata and in trichotillomania; hence the need for a differential diagnosis.

	1. Alopecia Areata	2. Trichotillomania
Definition	Hair loss caused by immunological attack.	Traumatic hair loss caused by the subjects themselves.
Etiopathogenesis	Genetic predisposition, autoimmune pathogenesis.	Tic that involves rolling, rubbing, and pulling out the hair.
Time of onset	It may occur from the first months of life.	More common after the age of 5, though it can occur from age 2 years.
Number of patches	Single or multiple.	Usually single.
Diameter of patches	From 1 to 2 cm to total alopecia (loss of all hair).	From 3 to 4 cm up to 50% and more of the scalp.
Lesion morphology	Sharply demarcated, roundish.	Sharply demarcated, roundish or unnatural shape, i.e., square or S-shaped.
Hair within the alopecic patch	The patches are usually devoid of hair. At the periphery, "exclamation mark hair" may be present.	Hair is characteristically present, some of normal length, though most are broken and of variable length.
Eyelashes	Sometimes involved, particularly in total alopecia.	Rarely involved.
Dermoscopy	Exclamation mark hair, cadaverized hairs, pseudocomedones (Fig. 1b).	Broken hairs (Fig. 2b).

Diagnostic Summary

Alopecia areata: areas without hair, exclamation mark hair at the periphery.
Trichotillomania: history of tics; inside the patch, hair of different length can be found.

1. Alopecia Areata

2. Trichotillomania

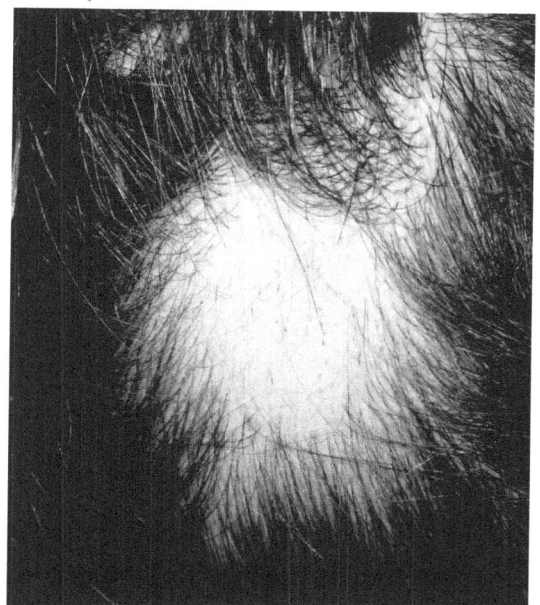

Fig. 1a

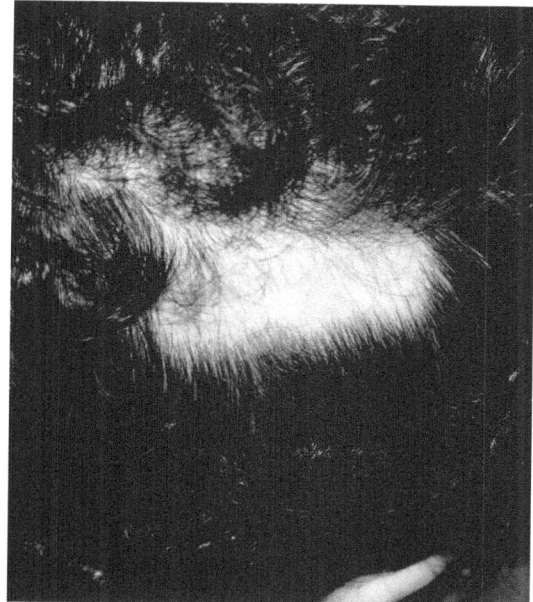

Fig. 2a

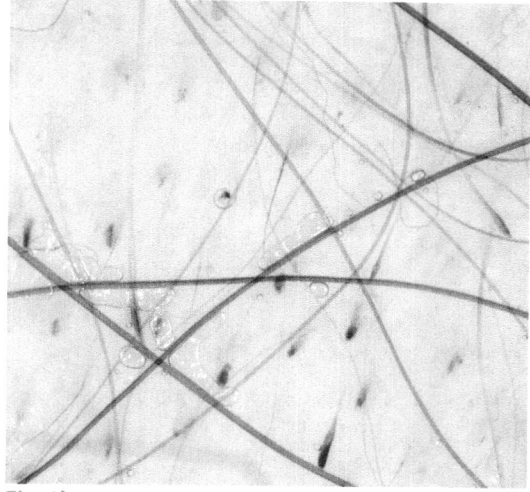

Fig. 1b

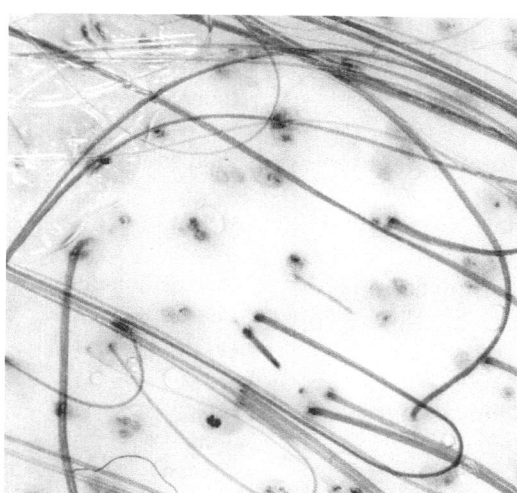

Fig. 2b

1. Alopecia Areata
2. Congenital Triangular Alopecia

Congenital triangular alopecia is a patch apparently devoid of hair, often localized to the frontal parietal region and shaped like an isosceles triangle with an anterior base, present early on in life and stable over time. Its early onset, persistence over time, and vaguely elongated shape are reminiscent of a nevus. In fact, it is also known as Brauer nevus [22]. Some authors [23] showed that the apparently alopecic area of congenital triangular alopecia really has a normal density of hair, although it is very thin vellus hair. This condition must be differentiated from alopecia areata.

	1. Alopecia Areata	2. Congenital Triangular Alopecia
Definition	Autoimmune disease characterized by hair loss leaving round, bald patches.	Localized patch resembling a nevus, possessing miniaturized hair.
Time of onset	Any age.	Present at birth or from early on in life, it sometimes becomes apparent in older age.
Subjective symptoms	Sometimes itching.	Absent.
Shape	Roundish.	Often triangular.
Number of patches	From one to dozens.	Single or double.
Hair	Absent.	Miniaturized.
Dermoscopy	Exclamation mark hair (Fig. 1b), pseudocomedones, and cadaverized hair.	Thin, poorly pigmented hair (Fig. 2b).
Clinical course	The patches tend to become larger at the periphery, may heal spontaneously or gradually extend, but never stay with the same extension over time.	The patch remains unchanged over time.

Diagnostic Summary

Alopecia areata: it is devoid of hair and changes over time.
Congenital triangular alopecia: it presents vellus hair and remains unchanged over time.

1. Alopecia Areata

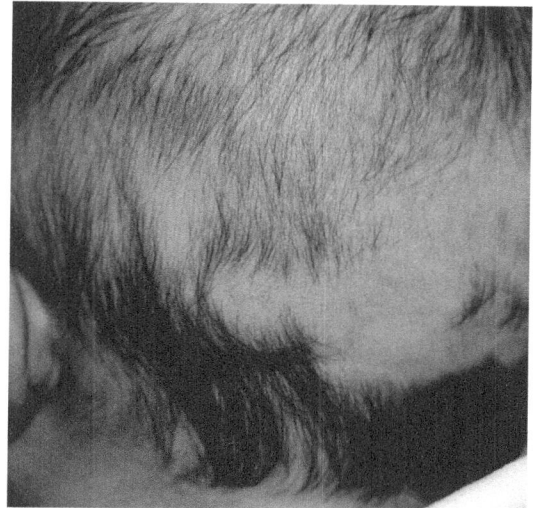

Fig. 1a

2. Congenital Triangular Alopecia

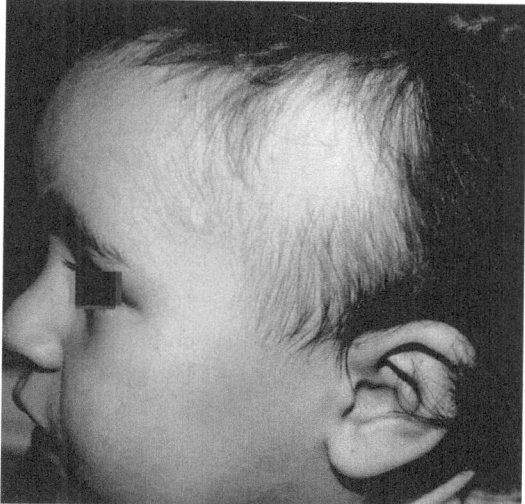

Fig. 2a

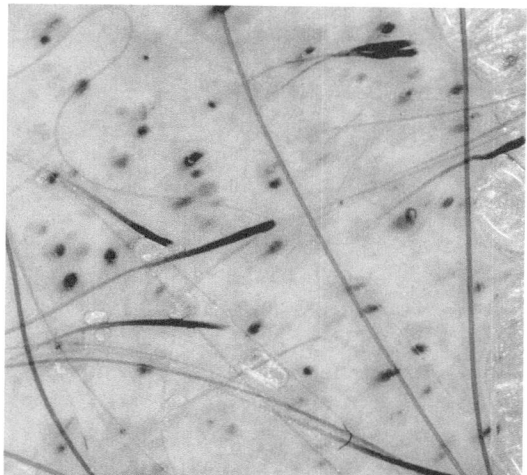

Fig. 1b Dermoscopy: exclamation mark hair

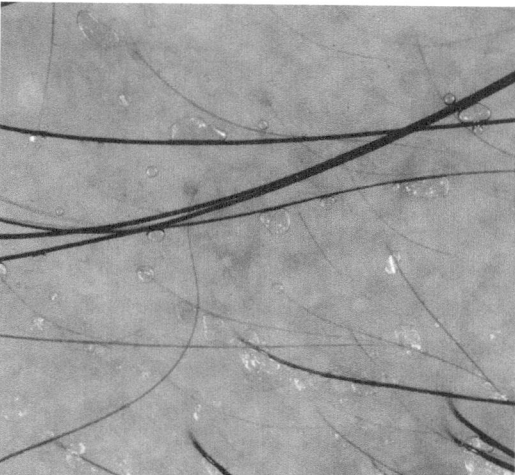

Fig. 2b Dermoscopy: thin and hypopigmented hair

1. Vitiligo
2. Genital Lichen Sclerosus

Vitiligo and lichen sclerosus are quite easily distinguishable from a clinical point of view. Problems can arise when they are localized exclusively to the genital region, where the white coloration of lichen sclerosus can be confused with that of vitiligo.

	1. Vitiligo	2. Genital Lichen Sclerosus
Definition	Autoimmune disease that causes the destruction of melanocytes.	Autoimmune disease that causes sclerosis of the superficial dermis.
Exclusive involvement of the genital region	Rare but possible, especially in focal vitiligo.	Frequent.
Symptoms	Absent.	Burning sensation when erosions are present; dysuria due to inflammation or stenosis of the external urethral meatus.
Lesion outline	Regular.	Sometimes irregular due to the presence of peripheral isolated micropapules.
Affected sites	In females, the labia majora (outer labia) and perivulvar skin; in males, the foreskin, penis, and scrotum.	In females, the labia majora and labia minora (inner labia). In males, the glans penis and around the external urethral meatus, which may be stenotic.
Surface appearance	Uniformly white with normal skin texture.	Varied because of the possible presence of hemorrhages (Figs 2a, 2b), erosions, epidermal atrophy.
Prognosis	It tends to persist and can extend.	It can improve during puberty, persist indefinitely, or evolve into a squamous cell carcinoma in adults.
Response to immunosuppressive therapy	Sometimes it responds to powerful corticosteroids, though usually transiently.	It responds very well, though transiently, to topical immunosuppressive therapy, both with corticosteroids and tacrolimus [24].

1. Vitiligo

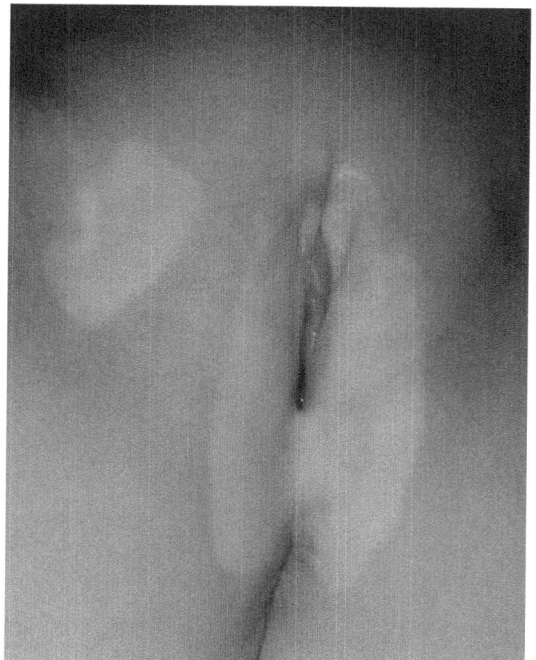

Fig. 1a

2. Genital Lichen Sclerosus

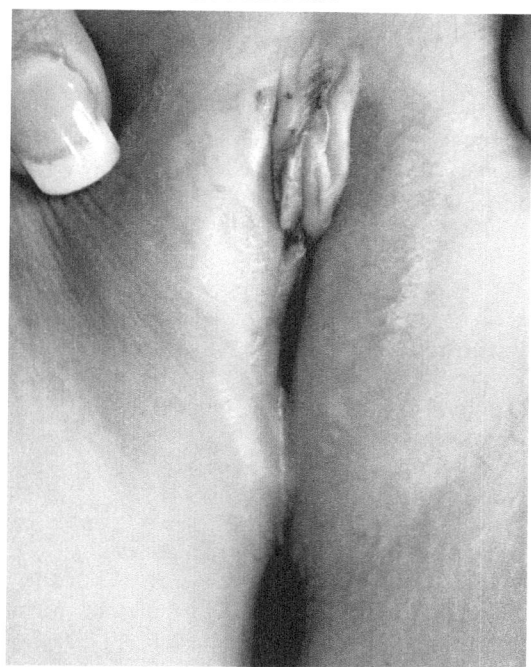

Fig. 2a

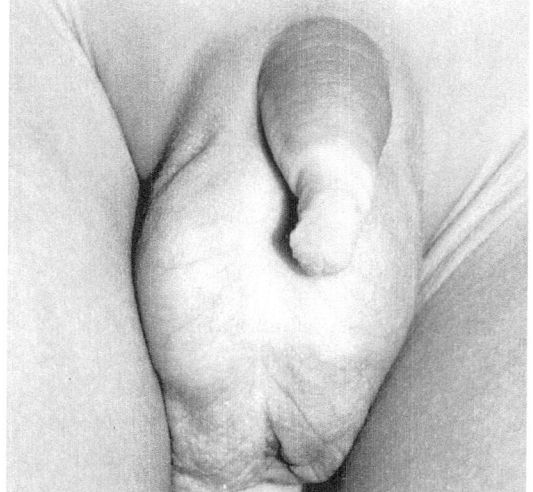

Fig. 1b

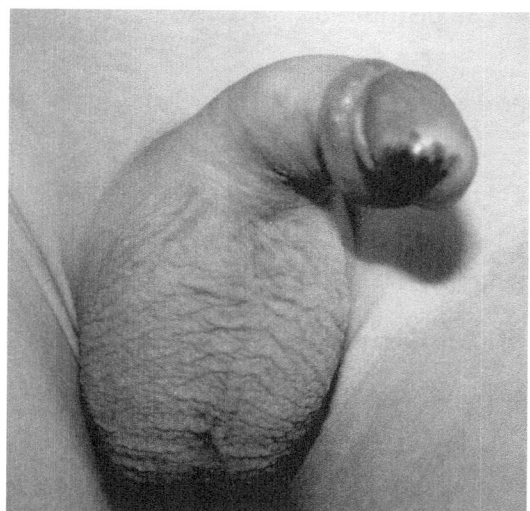

Fig. 2b

Diagnostic Summary

Vitiligo: no subjective symptoms; it has uniformly white coloration and responds poorly to immunosuppressive therapy.

Genital lichen sclerosus: subjective symptoms; it has variegated coloration due to the presence of hemorrhages and responds better to topical immunosuppressive therapy.

1. Lichen Planus
2. Lichen Aureus

Despite the similar name, lichen planus and lichen aureus are two different diseases. The former is an autoimmune disease, while the latter is a capillaritis of uncertain etiopathogenesis [25]. When only skin pigmentation findings are available, the differential diagnosis between the two diseases can be particularly difficult, though dermoscopy can be a useful diagnostic tool in this instance.

	1. Lichen Planus	2. Lichen Aureus
Pathogenesis	Autoimmune.	Unknown.
Mucosal involvement	Frequent.	Absent.
Nail involvement	Possible.	Absent.
Itching	Often present.	Rare.
Skin lesions	Flat papules and pigmented sequelae.	Flat papules and pigmented maculae.
Type of pigment	Melanin.	Hemosiderin.
Lesion distribution	Usually bilateral, rarely segmental.	Usually segmental, rarely bilateral.
Primary location	Volar surface of the wrists, limbs, chest.	Lower limbs.
Color of pigmented lesions	Purplish or sepia.	Red-brownish or sepia.
Red dots	Never.	Always, except during remission.
Disease duration	Usually less than 1 year.	Usually, more than 2 years.
Dermoscopy	Pearly-white, amorphous, branched structures, at the periphery of which hyperpigmented red-brownish thin tips, parallel or radial, and globules can be seen (Fig. 1b).	Greater or lesser number of red globules, with blurred borders, which stand out against a brownish background (Fig. 2b).
Histological findings	Hypergranulosis, vacuolar degeneration of the cells of the basal layer, sawtooth epidermal crests, band-like lymphocytic infiltrate in the superficial dermis.	Band-like lymphocytic infiltrate in the superficial dermis, edematous endothelial cells and dilated capillaries, extravasated erythrocytes and hemosiderin pigment.

1. Lichen Planus

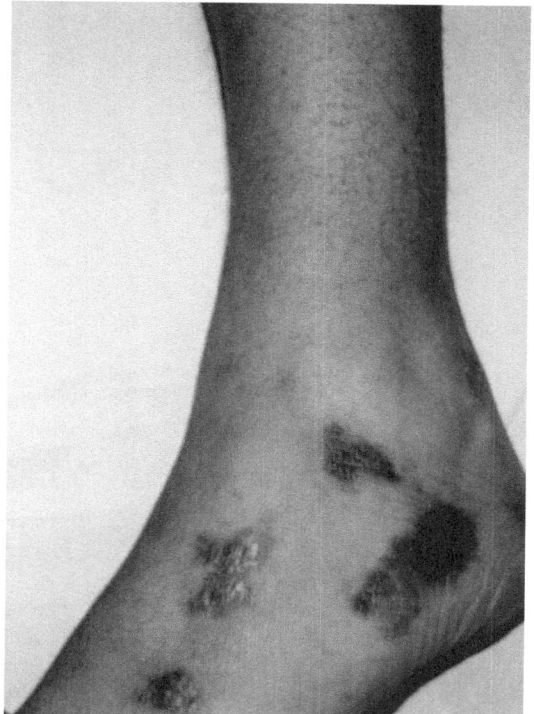

Fig. 1a

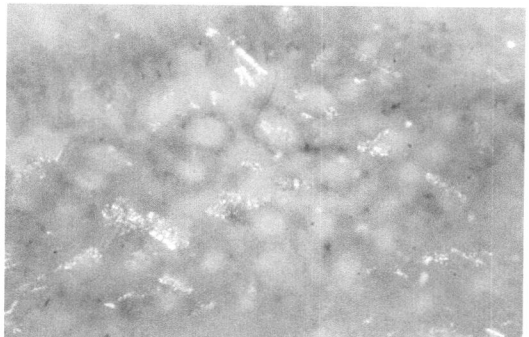

Fig. 1b Dermoscopy of Fig. 1a

2. Lichen Aureus

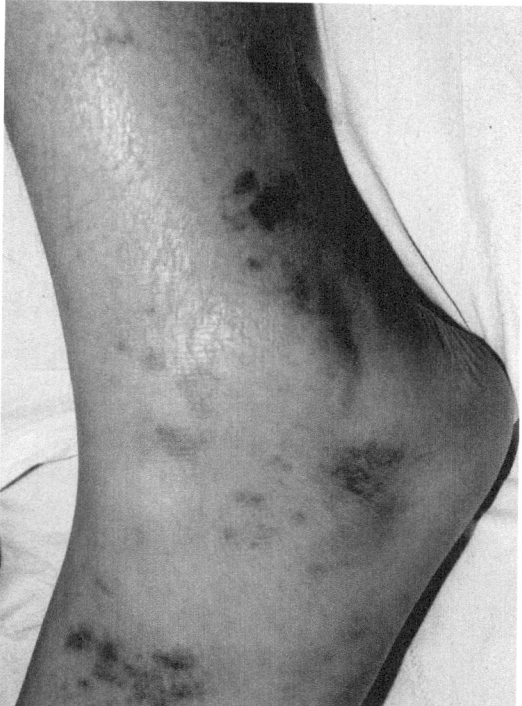

Fig. 2a

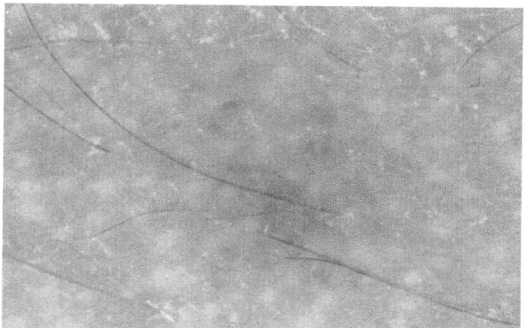

Fig. 2b Dermoscopy of Fig. 2a

Diagnostic Summary

Lichen planus: no red globules present.
Lichen aureus: red globules are visible to the naked eye, more so using a dermoscope.

Miscellaneous Items

E. Bonifazi, *Differential Diagnosis in Pediatric Dermatology,*
DOI: 10.1007/978-88-470-2859-3_10 © Springer-Verlag Italia 2013

1. Plantar Ecchymosis
2. Plantar Melanocytic Nevus

Sometimes, a plantar bruise can simulate a melanocytic nevus. The clinical history of the patient does not always clarify the time of onset.

	1. Plantar Ecchymosis	2. Plantar Melanocytic Nevus
Age involved	More common in young athletic subjects.	Any age.
History	An ecchymosis of 6–7 mm cannot last for more than 3 months. A history of trauma can be detected.	A nevus of 6 mm or larger must have a history lasting several years and could not have been noticed only in the last month or so.
Symmetry	Usually unilateral, it may be bilateral and symmetrical (Fig. 1a).	Usually unilateral.
Irregular coloration	Absent.	Sometimes present.
Dermoscopy	Blood lacunae; when superficial, they are distributed along the dermatoglyphics (Fig. 1b).	Melanin pigment; when superficial, it is distributed along the furrows (Fig. 2b).
Clinical course	Intraepidermal ecchymoses reach the surface within several weeks and are then eliminated as squamous crusts.	Melanocytic nevi persist unchanged over time, regardless of the slow growth due to the progressive lengthening of the foot in children.

Diagnostic Summary

Plantar ecchymosis: blackish lesions appear suddenly, with blood lacunae on dermoscopy.
Plantar melanocytic nevus: persistent blackish lesion with melanocytic pattern on dermoscopy.

1. Plantar Ecchymosis

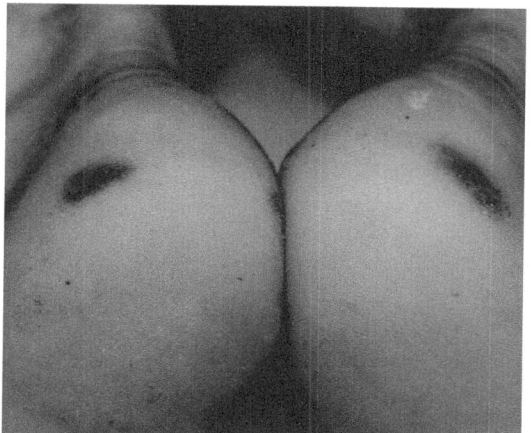

Fig. 1a

2. Plantar Melanocytic Nevus

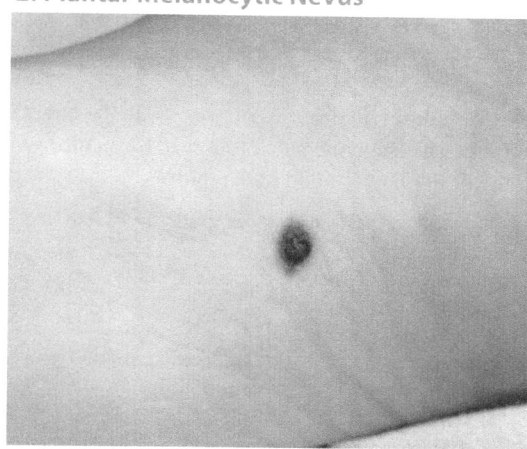

Fig. 2a

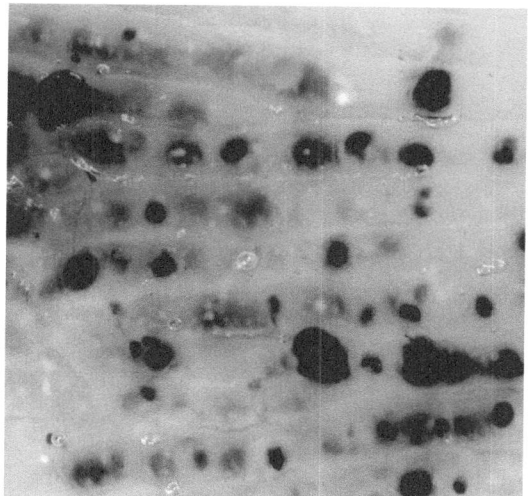

Fig. 1b Dermoscopy of Fig. 1a with blood lacunae

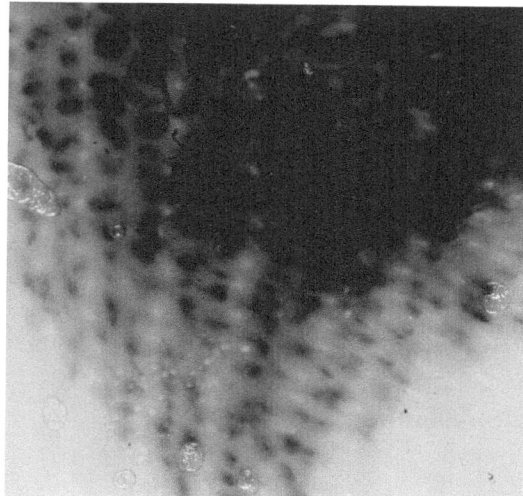

Fig. 2b Dermoscopy of Fig. 2a with melanocytic pattern

1. Gangrene of the Buttock
2. Hemangioma

Two very different diseases may occur in the buttock of the neonate, which share very similar clinical features, i.e., an ischemic patch followed by an ulcer with clearly defined borders: these two diseases are gangrene of the buttock and hemangioma.

	1. Gangrene of the Buttock	2. Hemangioma
Definition	Necrosis caused by arterial occlusion.	Benign tumor of angiopoietic cells.
Time of onset	At birth.	First few days of life.
Initial lesion	More or less extensive ischemic patch, depending on the level of arterial occlusion.	More or less extensive (3–6 cm) ischemic patch, sometimes with central telangiectasias.
Duration of ischemic patch	Minutes.	Hours or days.
Associated disorders	Persistent palsy of the sciatic nerve.	None.
Subsequent skin lesions	Deep, blackish necrosis, followed by eschar detachment and ulceration.	Erosion followed by ulceration; hemangiomatous foci at the periphery of the ulcer.
Ulcer depth	1–3 cm.	2–3 mm.

Diagnostic Summary

Gangrene of the buttock: necrosis and deep ulceration with palsy of the sciatic nerve occur following ischemia that lasts only a few minutes.
Hemangioma: after ischemia lasting for hours or days, sometimes with telangiectasias, a superficial ulcer appears; at its periphery, hemangiomatous foci are visible.

1. Gangrene of the Buttock

2. Hemangioma

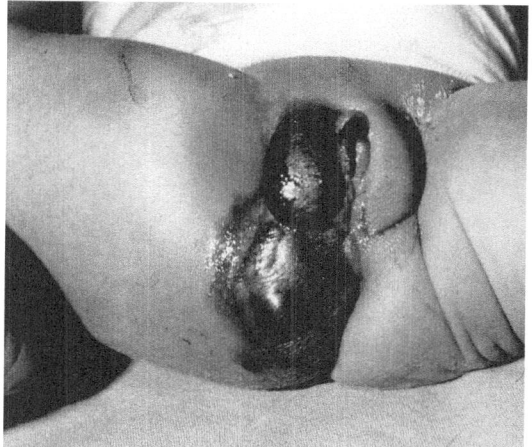

Fig. 1a Vulvar and gluteal gangrene

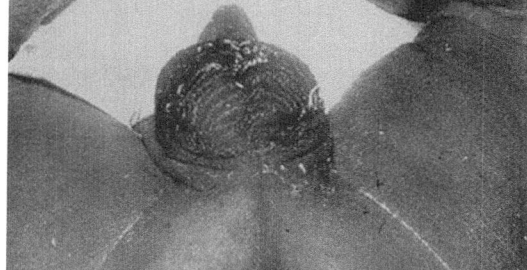

Fig. 2a Precursor of hemangioma at birth

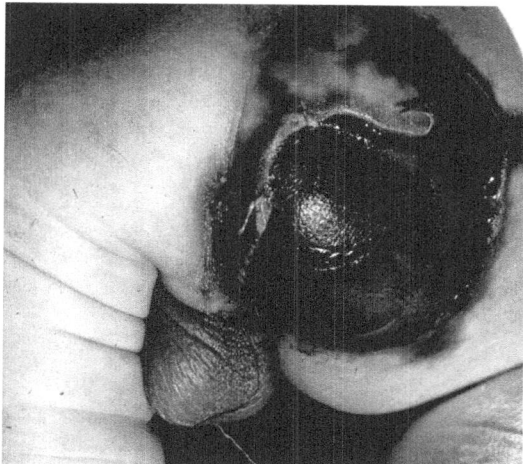

Fig. 1b Gluteal gangrene in infant aged 7 days

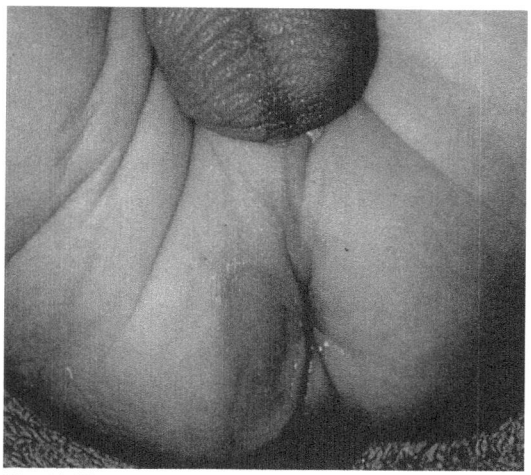

Fig. 2b The same child as in Fig. 2a presenting with ulcer at the age of 7 days

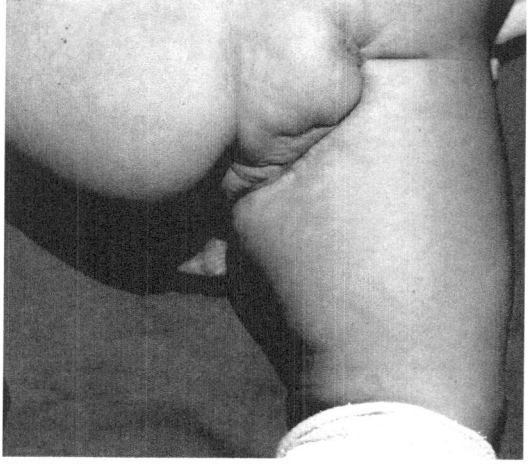

Fig. 1c Same patient as in Fig. 1b with scar at the age of 40 days

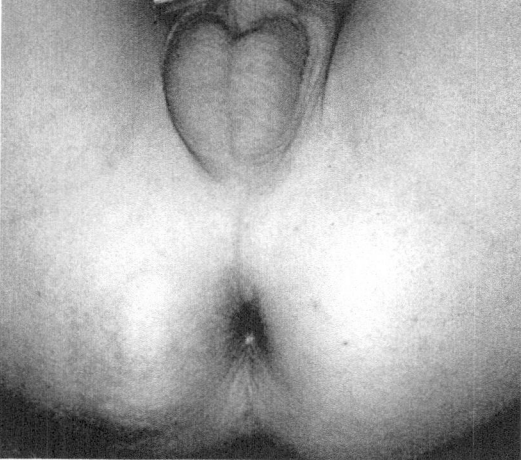

Fig. 2c Same patient as in Fig. 2a and 2b with scar at the age of 2 months

1. Knuckle Pads
2. Finger Biting Tic

Finger biting tic should be differentiated from knuckle pads, a rare fibromatosis affecting the hands [26].

	1. Knuckle Pads	**2. Finger Biting Tic**
Definition	Fibromatosis of the dorsum of the phalanges in the periarticular region.	Tic.
Location	Proximal interphalangeal joints, sometimes the metacarpophalangeal and distal interphalangeal joints.	Dorsal surface of the hands and/or fingers.
Number of lesions	Multiple, bilateral, evenly distributed.	Single or multiple.
Time of onset	Adolescents and young adults.	Young adults, rarely children.
Pathogenetic mechanism	Idiopathic.	Compulsive rubbing, pinching, and chewing.

Diagnostic Summary

Knuckle pads: multiple lesions regularly distributed on the dorsal surface of the small joints of the hands.
Finger biting tic: a single or double irregular nodule of the hand in a subject with history of biting.

1. Knuckle Pads

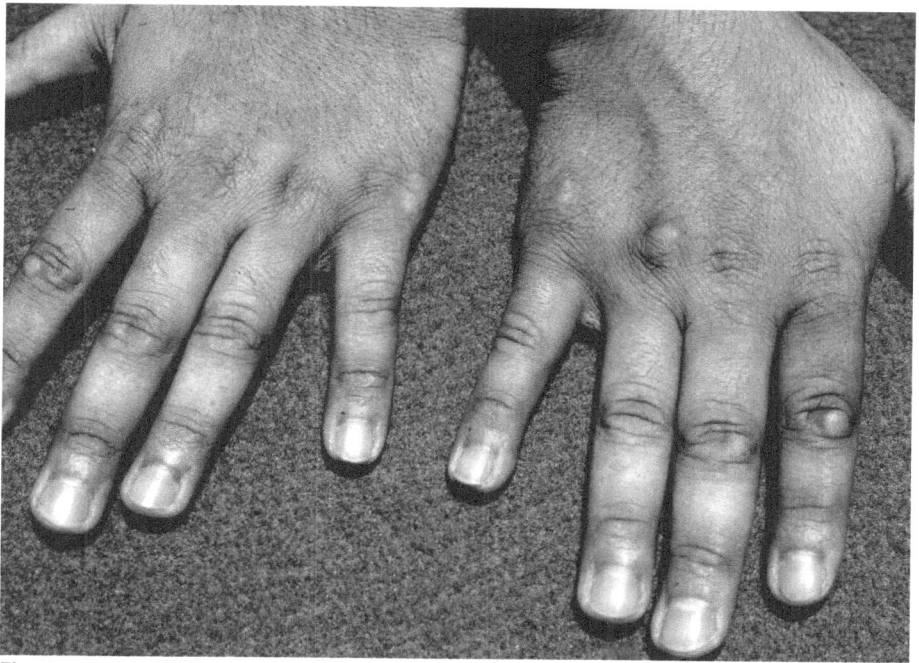

Fig. 1

2. Finger Biting Tic

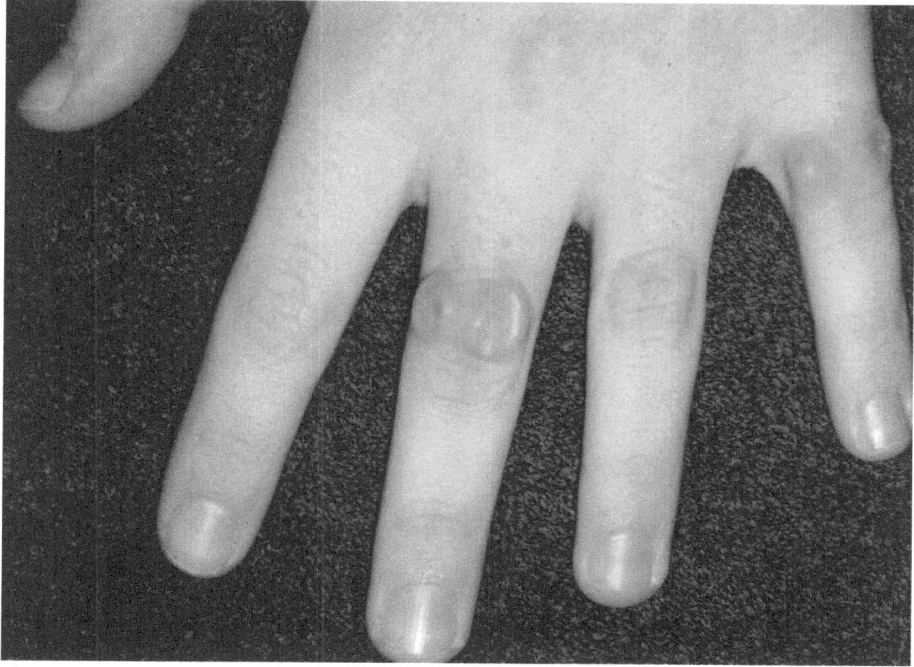

Fig. 2

Connective Tissue Diseases

E. Bonifazi, *Differential Diagnosis in Pediatric Dermatology,*
DOI: 10.1007/978-88-470-2859-3_11 © Springer-Verlag Italia 2013

1. Systemic Lupus Erythematosus
2. Dermatomyositis

Both systemic lupus erythematosus and dermatomyositis may present with a facial heliotrope rash, thereby requiring a differential diagnosis.

	1. Systemic Lupus Erythematosus	2. Dermatomyositis
Definition	Connective tissue disease characterized by the involvement of many organs and by immunological abnormalities.	Connective tissue disease characterized by a predominant muscle and skin involvement [27].
Juvenile characteristics	Not relevant.	Systemic vasculitis and increased incidence of calcification; no association with malignancy.
Incidence in the first decade	Rare.	Frequent.
Difference between the sexes	The female/male ratio is 8:1 in the peripubertal period.	The disease is twice more frequent in females.
Face	Heliotrope erythema affecting the cheeks and bridge of the nose.	Heliotrope erythema and "lilac" edema of the eyelids.
Hands	Periungual erythema and telangiectasias.	Gottron papules on the dorsal, metacarpophalangeal joints.
Systemic involvement	Fever, arthralgia, and nephritis are the most frequent findings.	Muscular weakness.
Laboratory findings	Leukopenia, elevated erythrocyte sedimentation rate, hematuria, hypocomplementemia, and anti-native DNA antibodies.	Increased serum creatine phosphokinase, transaminases–especially glutamic-oxaloacetic transaminase–and lactate dehydrogenase.
Response to corticosteroids	Excellent.	Good.

Diagnostic Summary

Systemic lupus erythematosus: leukopenia, hypocomplementemia, anti-native DNA antibodies.

Dermatomyositis: Gottron papules, increased muscle enzymes.

1. Systemic Lupus Erythematosus

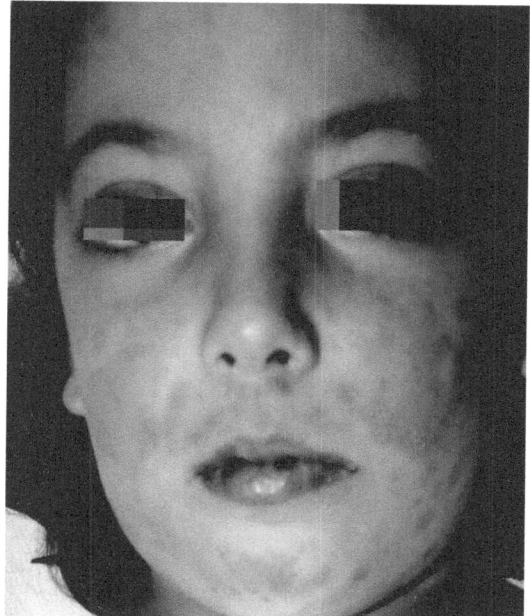

Fig. 1a

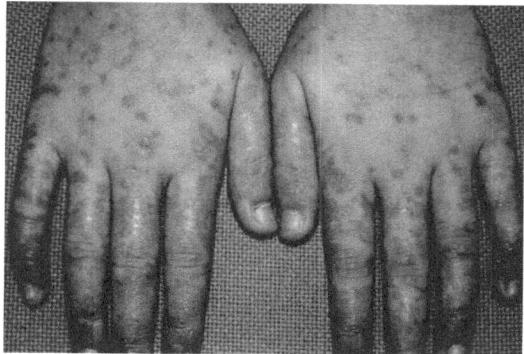

Fig. 1b

2. Dermatomyositis

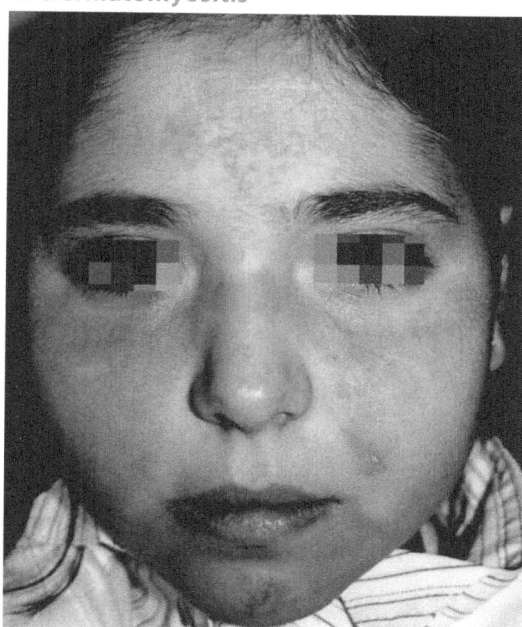

Fig. 2a

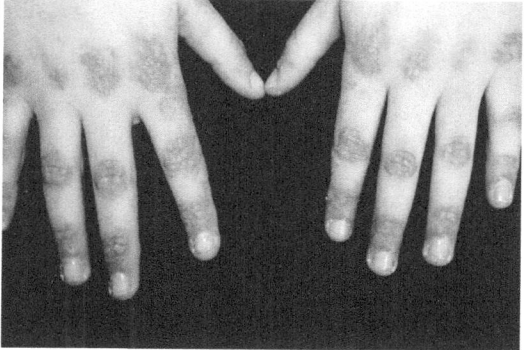

Fig. 2b

1. Systemic Lupus Erythematosus
2. Seborrheic Dermatitis

Erythematous lesions of the face may occur in adolescent girls both in systemic lupus erythematosus and seborrheic dermatitis, hence the usefulness of a differential diagnosis.

	1. Systemic Lupus Erythematosus	2. Seborrheic Dermatitis
Definition	Systemic autoimmune disease.	Constitutional dermatitis.
Difference between the sexes	Clearly prevalent in women of childbearing age.	No significant differences between the sexes.
Seasonality	It appears in late spring or summer and gets worse in the summer and with sun exposure.	It appears in spring or autumn and improves significantly in the summer.
Associated manifestations	Fever, arthralgia, anemia.	None, except sometimes acne.
Symptoms	None or mild burning sensation.	Sensation of "pulled skin".
Lesion location	Dorsal aspect of the nose and cheeks with a butterfly pattern.	Nasal alae, nasolabial grooves, cheeks, forehead.
Lesion type	Marked erythema.	Mild erythema and scaling.
Lesion persistence	Persist for a long time until the condition is diagnosed and treated.	Waxing and waning course with changes in days.
Non-facial lesions	Hands, periungual tissues.	Retroauricular and chest folds; midthoracic circinate lesions.
Laboratory findings	Increased nonspecific inflammatory markers (erythrocyte sedimentation rate, C-reactive protein levels), leukopenia, hypergamma-globulinemia, reduced C3 and C4, and presence of autoantibodies.	Within normal limits.

Diagnostic Summary

Systemic lupus erythematosus: persistent facial erythema that gets worse in the summer; alterations of other organs and laboratory findings.
Seborrheic dermatitis: facial erythema and scaling that improves in the summer; no alterations of other organs or laboratory findings.

1. Systemic Lupus Erythematosus

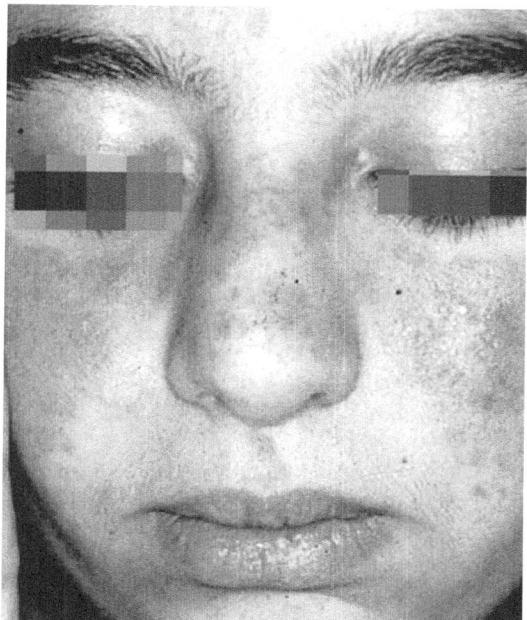

Fig. 1a

2. Seborrheic Dermatitis

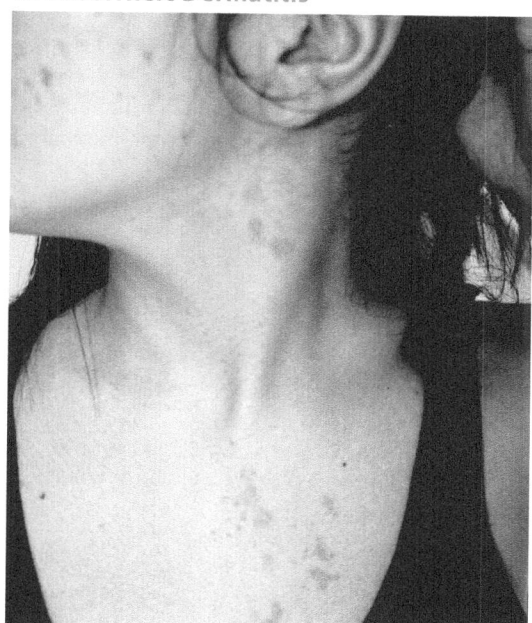

Fig. 2a

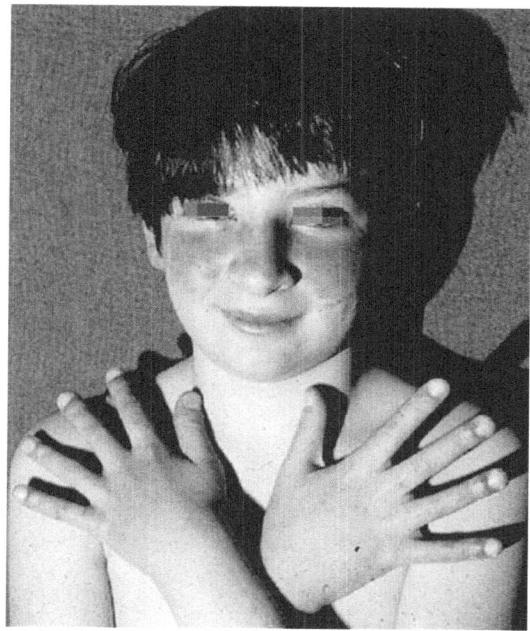

Fig. 1b

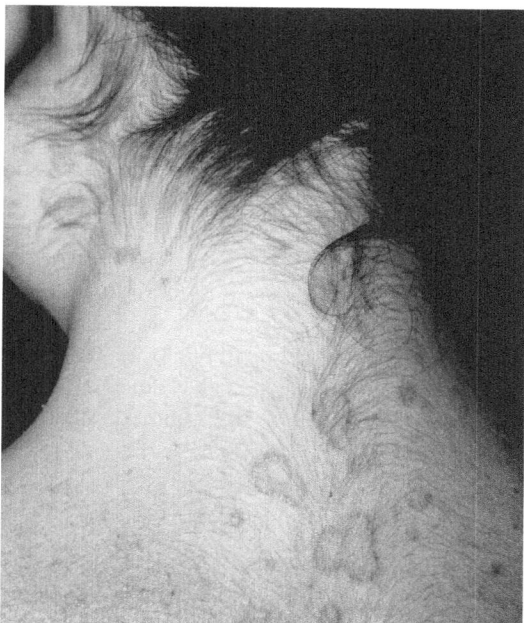

Fig. 2b

1. Initial Segmental Scleroderma
2. Unilateral Nevoid Telangiectasia

Segmental scleroderma in its initial inflammatory phase should be differentiated from unilateral nevoid telangiectasia, an acquired disorder reminiscent of a port-wine stain.

	1. Initial Segmental Scleroderma	2. Unilateral Nevoid Telangiectasia
Definition	Autoimmune skin disease localized in the dermis, which becomes sclerotic.	Acquired segmental telangiectasias due to an abnormal response to estrogens [28].
Difference between the sexes	Prevalent in females.	Prevalent in females.
Time of onset	First 3–4 decades.	Peripubertal.
Subjective symptoms	Sometimes, initial paresthesias.	Absent.
Lesion color	Pink, red, then porcelain-like.	Pink, red.
Clinical course	Sudden appearance of the erythema; after several weeks, progressive hardening and porcelain-like sclerosis starting from the center of the lesions. With time, regression of sclerosis with dyschromic and atrophic sequelae.	After the appearance of the first lesions, progression on the same segment of the initial lesions for several weeks. The skin disorder then remains unchanged throughout life.
Treatment	Immunosuppressive, though it does not significantly affect the clinical course of the disease.	Pulsed dye laser—585–595 nm— can induce lightening of the lesions.

Diagnostic Summary

Initial segmental scleroderma: inflammation without telangiectasias; the diagnosis becomes clearer with the appearance of the whitish sclerosis.
Unilateral nevoid telangiectasia: telangiectasias without inflammation.

1. Initial Segmental Scleroderma

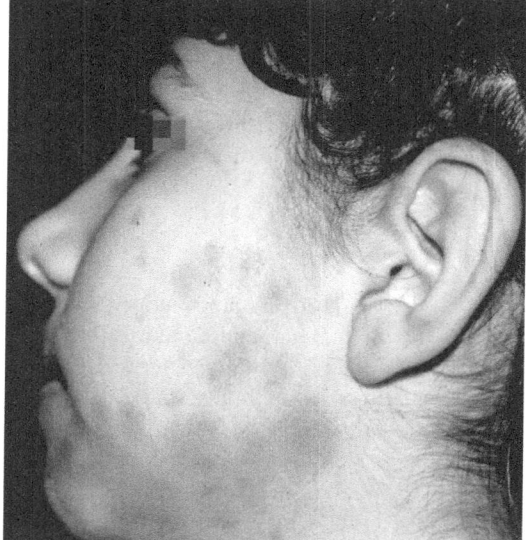

Fig. 1a

2. Unilateral Nevoid Telangiectasia

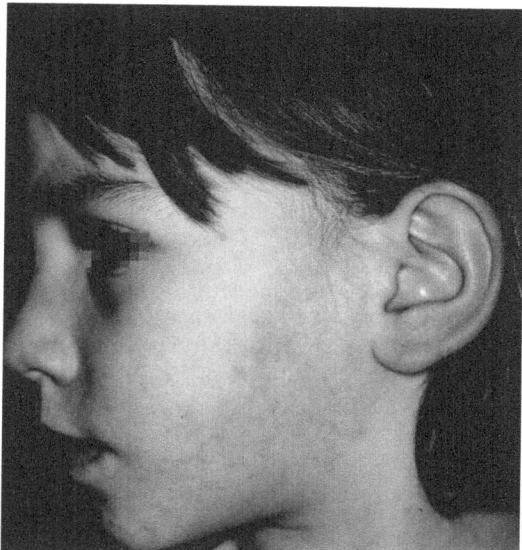

Fig. 2a

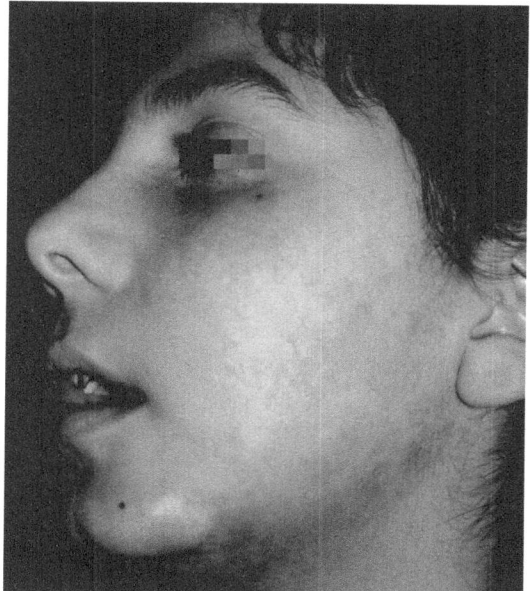

Fig. 1b Same girl as in Fig 1a with sclerosis on the chin

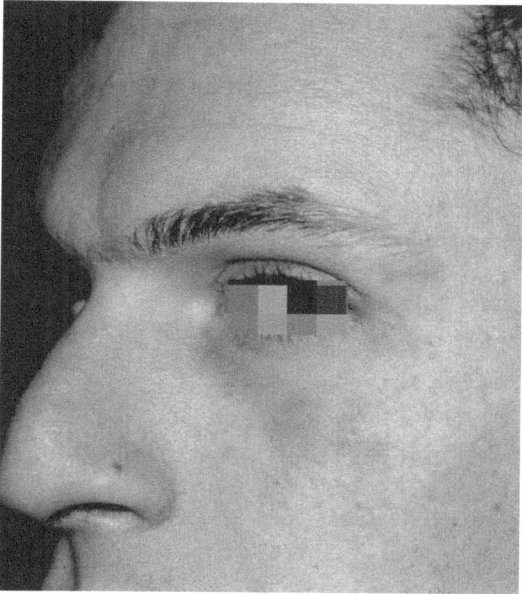

Fig. 2b

1. Gottron Papules
2. Plane Warts

The Gottron papules of dermatomyositis, when affecting exclusively or mainly the back of the hands, should be differentiated from plane warts, which need a different treatment. The differential diagnosis is even more difficult when plane warts on the back of the hands affect a patient with dermatomyositis.

	1. Gottron Papules	**2. Plane Warts**
Definition	Papular lesions due to inflammatory changes of the dermis.	Epidermal papules induced by human papillomavirus (HPV) infection and characterized by acanthosis and epidermal hyperkeratosis.
Location on the hands	Back of the hands, particularly at the level of the metacarpophalangeal and proximal interphalangeal joints.	Back of the hands without predilection for the surfaces covering the joints.
Lesion distribution	Symmetrical.	At least initially, they are more prevalent on one hand.
Other sites to be affected	Extensor surface of the elbows and knees.	Face.
Koebner phenomenon	Rare.	Frequent.
Other cutaneous findings	Heliotrope erythema, psoriasis-like lesions on the extensor surface of the elbows and knees.	None.
Other findings	Clinical and laboratory findings showing muscle involvement.	None.

Diagnostic Summary

Gottron papules: symmetrical and periarticular; they are associated with other signs of dermatomyositis.
Plane warts: initially asymmetrical without predilection for the joint surfaces.

1. Gottron Papules

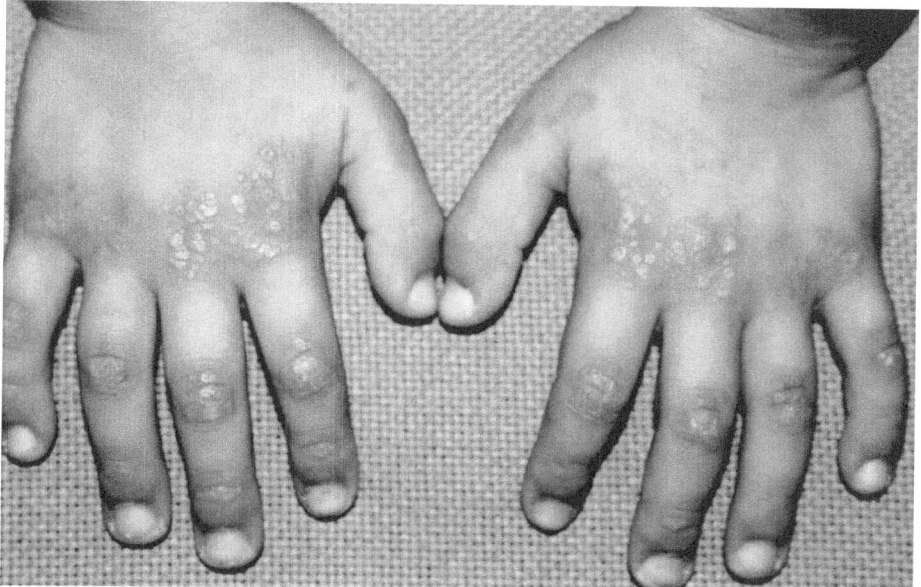

Fig. 1

2. Plane Warts

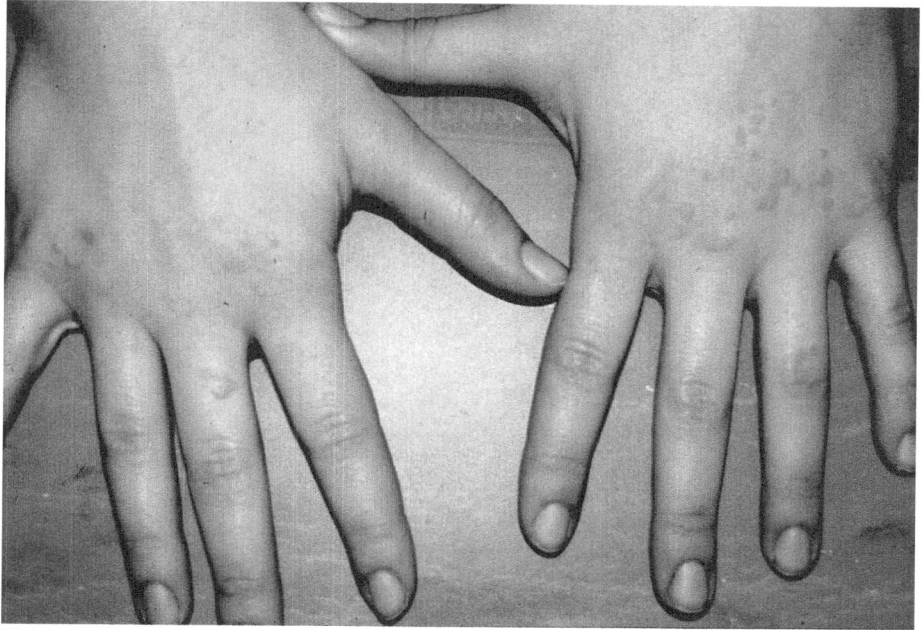

Fig. 2

Tumors

E. Bonifazi, *Differential Diagnosis in Pediatric Dermatology,*
DOI: 10.1007/978-88-470-2859-3_12 © Springer-Verlag Italia 2013

1. Pilomatricoma
2. Dermoid Cyst

Pilomatricoma can rarely become evident in the first months of life and therefore should be differentiated from a dermoid cyst.

	1. Pilomatricoma	2. Dermoid Cyst
Definition	Benign tumor that originates from the hair sheath.	Cyst containing epidermal remnants localized on the fusion lines.
Difference between the sexes	Prevalent in females.	No difference.
Time of onset	Any age; before 12 years of age in 42% of cases [29]; it very rarely occurs before the sixth month of life.	Usually present at birth or appearing in the first few months.
Number of lesions	Usually single, multiple in 5% of cases.	Single.
Site	Head, upper chest, upper limbs.	Head—lateral eyebrow, anterior fontanelle, glabella—neck, vertebral axis.
Color	Bluish, yellowish, red, skin-colored.	Skin-colored, rarely reddened.
Shape	Irregular surface, needle-shaped, spindle-shaped, in plaque.	Spherical with regular surface.

Diagnostic Summary

Pilomatricoma: variable color, irregular shape and surface.
Dermoid cyst: normal skin, regular surface, present in the perinatal period along the fusion lines.

1. Pilomatricoma

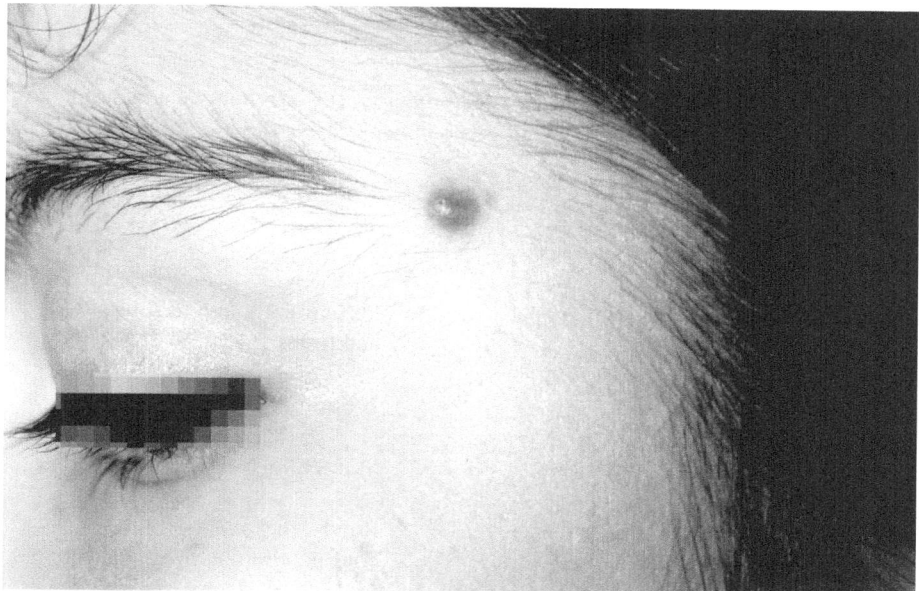

Fig. 1

2. Dermoid Cyst

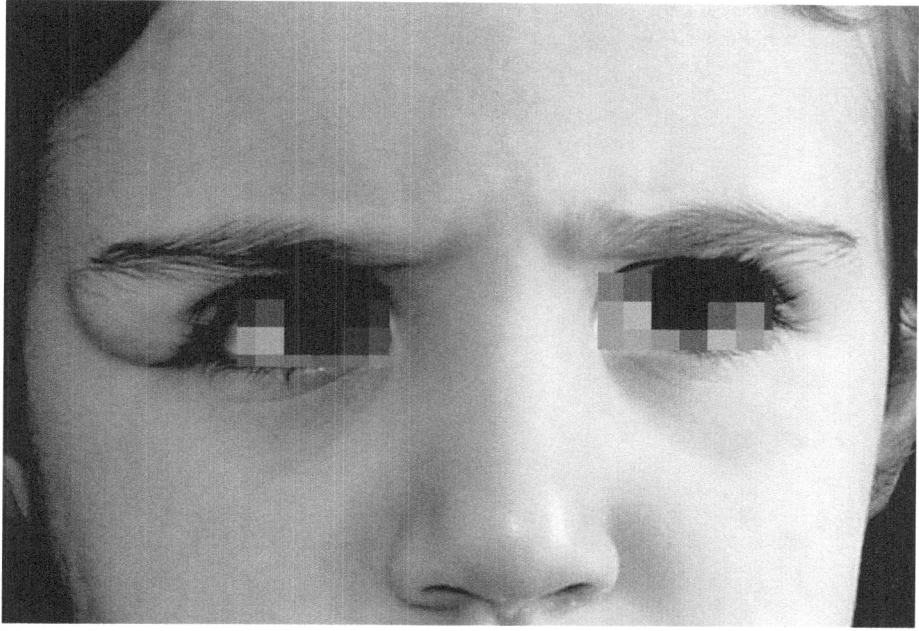

Fig. 2

1. Angiofibromas of Tuberous Sclerosis
2. Multiple Trichoepitheliomas

The clinical history and morphology of multiple trichoepitheliomas [30] can be reminiscent of the angiofibromas of tuberous sclerosis and therefore require a differential diagnosis.

	1. Angiofibromas of Tuberous Sclerosis	2. Multiple Trichoepitheliomas
Lesion location	Nasal and perinasal.	Perinasal, though the chest and limbs can be involved.
Lesion size	1–3 mm.	1–5 mm.
Color	Skin-colored or reddish.	Skin-colored or whitish.
Tendency to become confluent	Rare, even when lesions are very close one another.	Rarely, they can become confluent into large plaques.
Other skin findings	White patches, fibrous plaques, shagreen patch, Koenen tumors.	Absent.
Involvement of other organs	Seizures, cardiac rhabdomyoma, renal cysts.	Absent.

Diagnostic Summary

Angiofibromas of tuberous sclerosis: reddish color, other signs of tuberous sclerosis in the skin and other organs are present.
Multiple trichoepitheliomas: whitish color, no other signs in the skin and other organs.

1. Angiofibromas of Tuberous Sclerosis

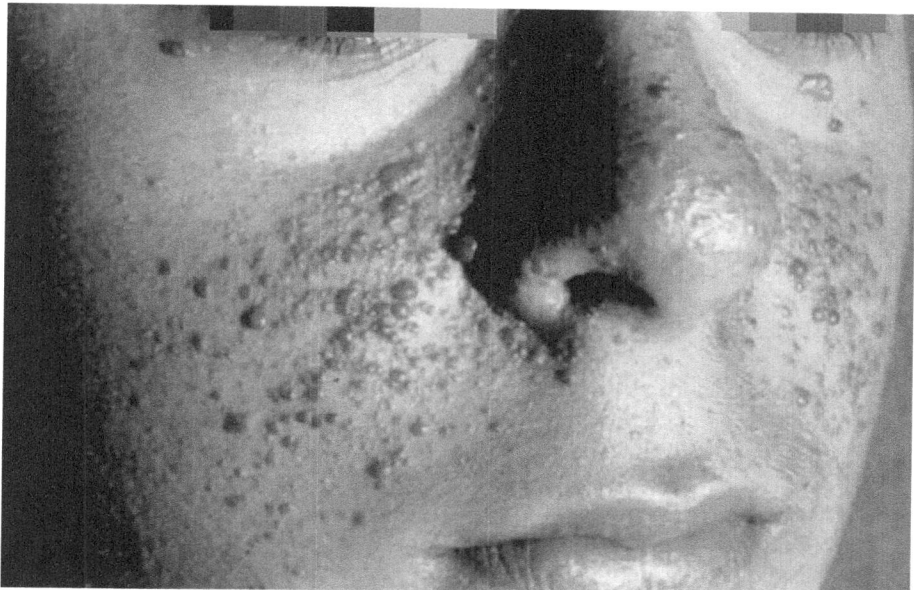

Fig. 1

2. Multiple Trichoepitheliomas

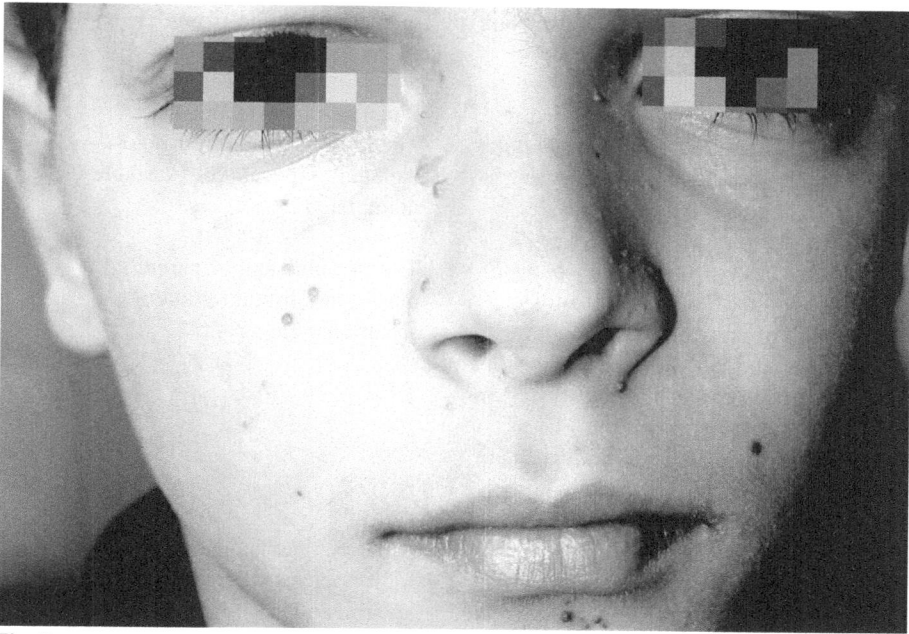

Fig. 2

1. Superficial Lymphangioma
2. Localized Angiokeratoma

Superficial lymphangioma and localized angiokeratoma are superficial, usually localized, vascular malformations. Although affecting the lymphatic vessels, lymphangioma characteristically undergoes intralesional hemorrhages. The latter can make the differential diagnosis from localized angiokeratoma difficult.

	1. Superficial Lymphangioma	2. Localized Angiokeratoma
Definition	It is a rare, stable, and localized malformation of the cutaneous lymphatic vessels. It can be associated with deep lymphangioma.	It is a rare malformation of the small, superficial blood vessels of the dermis with epidermal hyperplasia.
Elementary lesion	Translucent vesicle containing serous liquid. It is reminiscent of a frog's egg (Fig. 1a).	Erythema or red papule (Fig. 2a), which disappears or fades under finger pressure.
Lesion size	Vesicles can associate to form larger lesions of variable size, till they form blisters of several centimeters in diameter.	The lesions are characterized by a uniform or scarcely variable diameter, ranging from 0.5 to 2 mm.
Dermoscopy	Multilobulated appearance with whitish septa separating the lobules, sometimes with blood lacunae in their center (Fig. 1b).	Punctate blood lacunae. The latter are monomorphic, isolated, with scarcely variable diameter (Fig. 2b).
Lesion persistency	The frog-egg-like vesicles persist indefinitely. The largest lesions, which often contain blood, may appear suddenly, due to intralesional hemorrhage, which makes what was a virtual cavity a real one. They completely regress within weeks or months depending on their diameter.	The maculae and/or papules persist indefinitely without significant changes.
Morphological changes	They can occur only due to an intralesional hemorrhage, which can make pre-existing virtual cavities evident, with a blister or target-like appearance, or make previous serous vesicles red, with subsequent return to the initial appearance as soon as the blood spilled in the vesicle is reabsorbed.	Almost nonexistent, except for rare cases when epidermal erosion and crust formation occur.

1. Superficial Lymphangioma

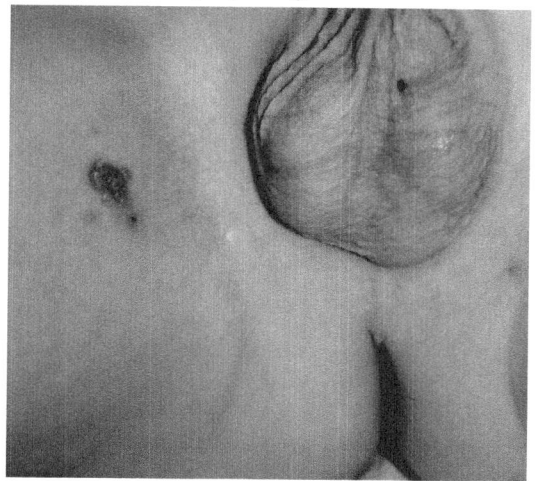

Fig. 1a

2. Localized Angiokeratoma

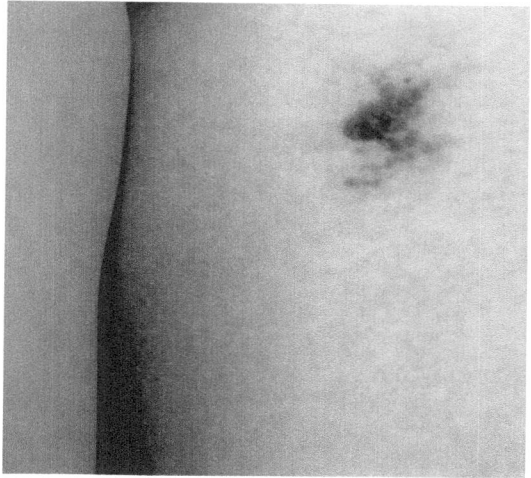

Fig. 2a

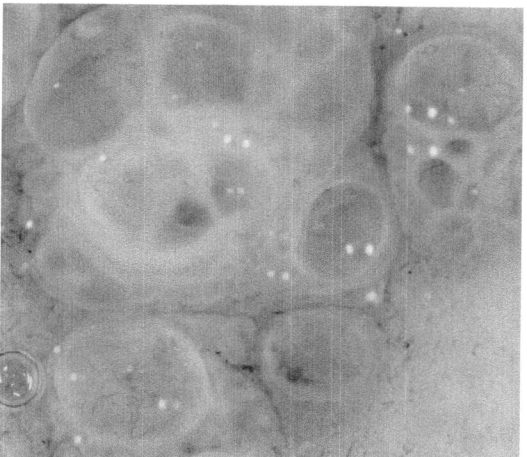

Fig. 1b Dermoscopy of Fig. 1a

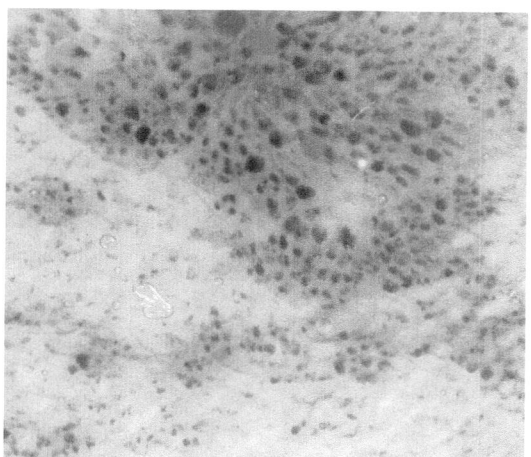

Fig. 2b Dermoscopy of Fig. 2a

Diagnostic Summary

Superficial lymphangioma: transiently, it takes on a reddish color due to intralesional hemorrhage.

Localized angiokeratoma: it is persistently red.

1. Keratosis Pilaris
2. Multiple Trichoepitheliomas

Keratosis pilaris is a disorder inherited as an autosomal dominant trait. It is characterized by hyperkeratosis of the follicular orifices, namely the external orifices of the pilosebaceous follicle.
Trichoepithelioma is a benign cutaneous tumor with primitive follicular differentiation. It is usually a solitary lesion, but multiple lesions can occur. The latter are inherited as an autosomal dominant trait [30].

	1. Keratosis Pilaris	2. Multiple Trichoepitheliomas
Definition	Inherited skin disorder characterized by hyperkeratosis of the follicular orifices.	Inherited skin disorder characterized by benign skin tumors with follicular differentiation.
Prevalence	1.1% of pediatric skin disorders [5].	Very rare.
Time of onset	Usually within the first year.	In 50% of cases, before the age of 6.
Summer improvement	Yes.	No.
Clinical course	It improves in decades.	Progressive worsening.
Surface	Rough.	Smooth.

Diagnostic Summary

Keratosis pilaris: lesions of uniform diameter, smaller than 1 mm, with summer improvement.
Multiple trichoepitheliomas: lesions ranging in diameter between 1 and 5 mm, sometimes translucent, without summer changes.

1. Keratosis Pilaris

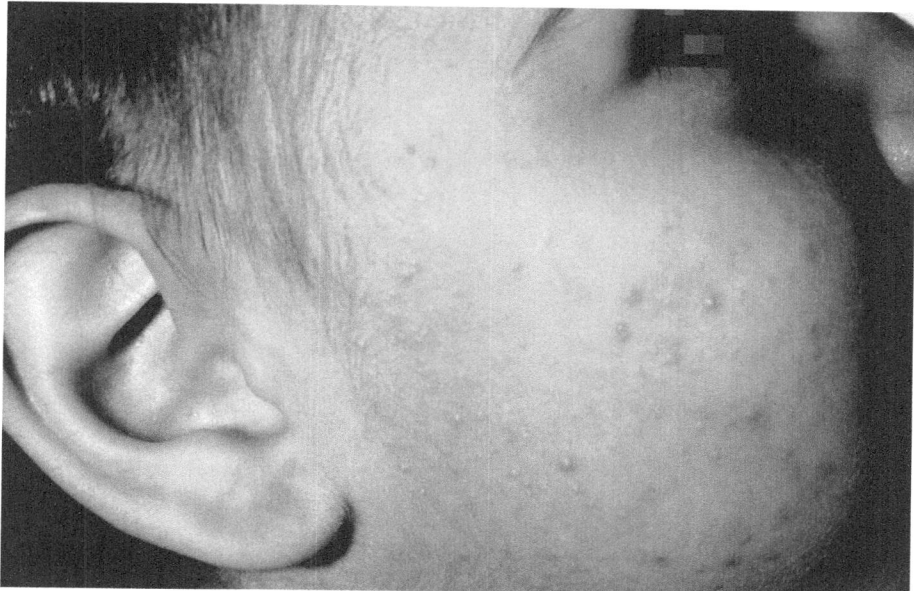

Fig. 1

2. Multiple Trichoepitheliomas

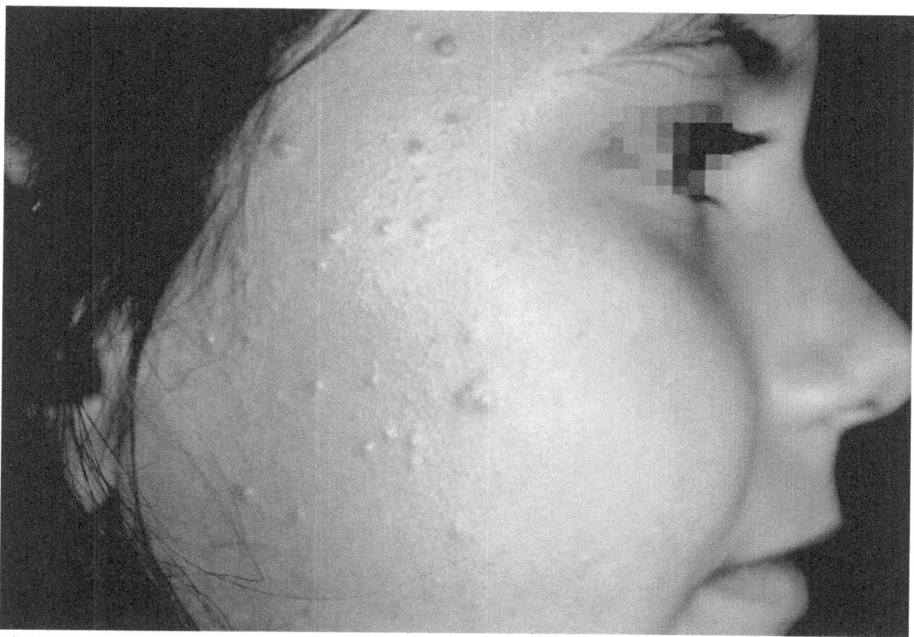

Fig. 2

References

1. Huson SM, Compston DAS, Clark P et al (1989) A genetic study of Von Recklinghausen neurofibromatosis in South East Wales. 1. Prevalence, fitness, mutation rate, and effect of parental transmissionon severity. J Med Genet 26:704–711
2. Chang A, Tung RC, Schlesinger T et al (2001) Familial cutaneous mastocytosis. Pediat Dermatol 18:271–276
3. Arakawa Y, Nakai N, Katoh N (2012) Rare case of basal cell carcinoma arising in a nevus sebaceous on the upper arm. J Dermatol. Jan 19. doi [Epub ahead of print]
4. Mazzotta F, Troccoli T, Petruzzelli V, Bonifazi E (1998) Role of capillary microscopy in the differential diagnosis of cutaneous angiomatous lesions of the newborn. Eur J Pediat Dermatol 8:89–92
5. Bonifazi E, Garofalo L, Meneghini CL (1981) Considerazioni epidemiologiche su 11.061 casi di dermatosi infantili. Dermatologia Clinica 1:87–94
6. Argenziano G, Agozzino M, Bonifazi E et al (2011) Natural evolution of Spitz nevi. Dermatology 222:256–260
7. Ahkami RN, Schwartz RA (1999) Nevus anemicus. Dermatology 198:327–329
8. Bonifazi E, Milano A, Caprio F, Garofalo L (2011) Hyperpigmented nevus. Eur J Pediat Dermatol 21:29–48
9. Bonifazi E, Milano A (2012) A new dermoscopic sign in juvenile xanthogranuloma. Eur J Pediat Dermatol 22:11–117
10. Müller CS, Schmaltz R, Vogt T, Pföhler C (2011) Lichen striatus and blaschkitis: reappraisal of the concept of blaschkolinear dermatoses. Br J Dermatol 164:257–262
11. Bonifazi E, Ciampo L (1999) Histiocytosis. Eur J Pediat Dermatol 9:417–432
12. Milano A, Bonifazi E (2012) Congenital melanocytic nevus. Clinical and dermoscopic signs of malignancy. Eur J Pediat Dermatol 22:135–143
13. Di Landro A, Grossi A, Pesenti G et al (2010) A scholastic out break of tinea due to trichophyton soudanense in Italy. Eur J Pediat Dermatol 20:227–230
14. Welch J (1998) Antenatal screening for syphilis (Editorial). BMJ 317:1605–1606
15. Patrizi A, Raone B, Neri I, D'Antuon A (2002) Infantile perianal protrusion. Pediatr Dermatol 19:15–18
16. Godoy Gijon E, Alonso San Pablo MT, Ruiz-Ayucar de la Vega I et al (2010) Scarlet fever variant of Staphylococcal scalded skin syndrome. An Pediatr (Barc) 72:434–435
17. França K, Villa RT, Silva IR et al (2011) Hair casts or pseudonits. Int J Trichology 3: 121–122
18. Foster RS, Bint LJ, Halbert AR (2012) Topical 0.1% rapamycin for angiofibromas in paediatric patients with tuberous sclerosis: a pilot study of four patients. Australas J Dermatol 53:52–56
19. Marqueling AL, Gilliam AE, Prendiville J et al (2006) Keratosis pilaris rubra: a common but underrecognized condition. Arch Dermatol 142:1611–1616
20. Coleman JC, Dobson NR (2006) Diagnostic dilemma: extremely low birth weight baby with staphylococcal scalded-skin syndrome or toxic epidermal necrolysis. J Perinatol 26:714–716
21. Garofalo L, Caprio F, Bonifazi E (1995) Psoriasis. Eur J Pediat Dermatol 5:129–144
22. García-Hernández MJ, Rodríguez-Pichardo A, Camacho F (1995) Congenital triangular alopecia (Brauer nevus). Pediatr Dermatol 12:301–303
23. Trakimas C, Sperling LC, Skelton HG et al (1994) Clinical and histologic findings in temporal triangular alopecia. J Am Acad Dermatol 31:205–209

24. Chi CC, Kirtschig G, Baldo M et al (2012) Systematic review and meta-analysis of ran-domized controlled trials on topical interventions for genital lichen sclerosus. J Am Acad Dermatol 67:305–312
25. Finch-Puches R, Wolf P, Kerl H, et al (2008) Lichen aureus. Arch Dermatol 144:1169–1173
26. Nenoff P, Woitek G (2011) Knuckle pads. N Eng J Med 364:2451
27. Kishi T, Miyamae T, Hara R et al (2012) Clinical analysis of 50 children with juvenile dermatomyositis. Mod Rheumatol Apr 22 [Epub ahead of print]
28. Guedes R, Leite L (2012) Unilateral nevoid telangectasia: a rare disease? Indian J Dermatol 57:138–140
29. Bonifazi E, Tarantino G (2000) Epidermal and adnexal tumors. Eur J Pediat Dermatol 10: 465–480
30. Manchanda K, Bansal M., Bhayana AA et al (2012) Brooke-Spiegler syndrome: a rare entity. Int J Trichology 4:29–31

Index

The manufacturer's authorised representative in the EU is Springer
Nature Customer Service Centre GmbH, Europaplatz 3, 69115 Heidelberg,
Germany. If you have any concerns regarding our products, please
contact ProductSafety@springernature.com

Printed and bound by CPI Group (UK) Ltd, Croydon, CR0 4YY

29/04/2026

02099458-0020